Gentle Yoga for Healing

Mind Body Spirit

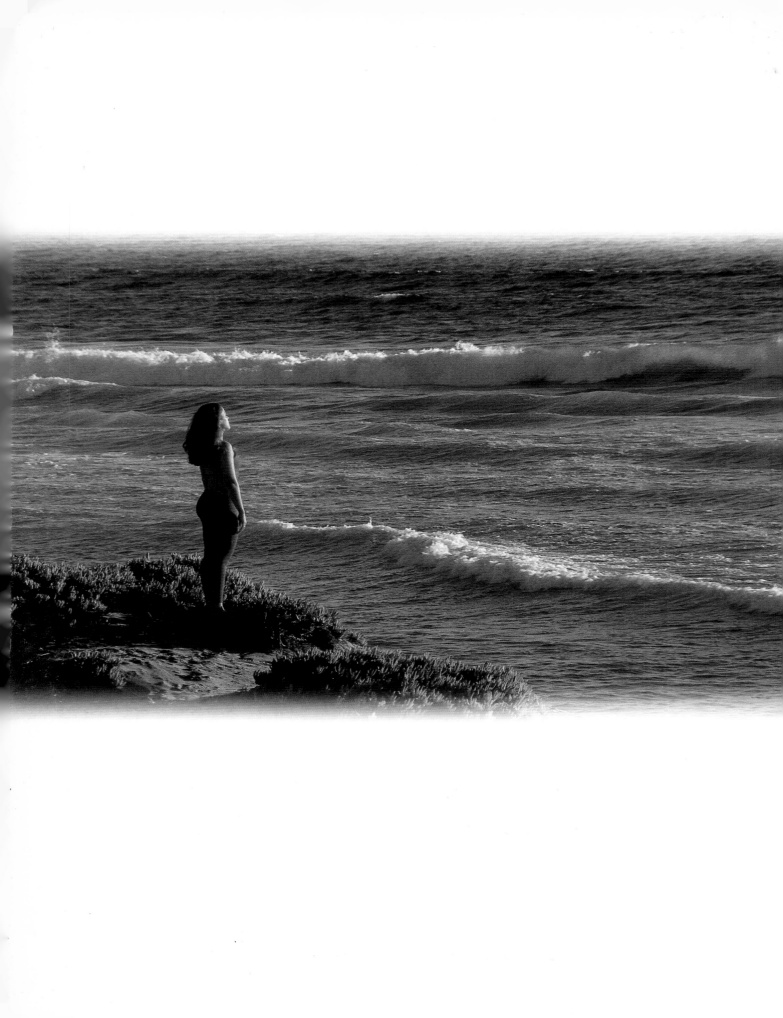

Gentle Yoga
for Healing
Mind
Body
Spirit

ANNALISA CUNNINGHAM

Photography by Dennis Burkhart

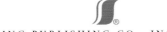

STERLING PUBLISHING CO., INC. NEW YORK

Acquisition, editing, and packaging by Diane Asay

Art direction and design by Lubosh Cech
www.okodesignstudio.com

Photography by Dennis Burkhart

This book is not intended to replace expert medical advice. The author and the publisher urge you to verify the appropriateness of any procedure or exercise with your qualified health care professional. The author and the publisher disclaim any liability or loss, personal or otherwise, resulting from the procedures and information in this book.

Library of Congress Cataloging-in-Publication Data Available

10 9 8 7 6 5 4 3 2 1

Published by Sterling Publishing Co., Inc.
387 Park Avenue South, New York, N.Y. 10016
© 2003 by Annalisa Cunningham
Distributed in Canada by Sterling Publishing
C/o Canadian Manda Group, One Atlantic Avenue, Suite 105
Toronto, Ontario, Canada M6K 3E7
Distributed in Great Britain by Chrysalis Books
64 Brewery Road, London N7 9NT, England
Distributed in Australia by Capricorn Link (Australia) Pty. Ltd.
P.O. Box 704, Windsor, NSW 2756, Australia

Sterling ISBN 0-8069-4584-2

Acknowledgments

Writing a book is a journey that involves many people along the way. I begin by thanking all of the yoga students who have participated in my classes throughout the years as a part of their own healing process. Without you, this work would have no purpose.

As a student of yoga I am forever grateful for the guidance and wealth of information given to me by the yoga teachers I have studied with. Your inspiration has touched my life in miraculous ways.

The actual creation of this book was birthed by a wonderful crew. Many thanks are due to Diane Asay, my editor, who valued this book from its conception; to Lubosh Cech, talented and creative designer, and to Dennis Burkhart, superb photographer who gave 100% plus to the project.

Special thanks to Dr. Myron Wentz for creating such a beautiful and healing environment at Sanoviv Medical Institute, and for his willingness to let us photograph there. A warm thanks to Kim Ward and Hilary Stokes for their wonderful assistance and photo modeling while we were at Sanoviv; and to models Mariella Lizarraga, Ricardo Perez, David Gonzalez, and Rosa Perez. We couldn't have asked for a nicer group of people to work with.

I'd also like to acknowledge models Akana Ma, Kelly Jones, Barry Shulak, and Jan Burkhart for their time at the studio in Portland. In addition I extend a heartfelt thanks to Dennis, Jan, Galen and Amber Burkhart for their wonderful hospitality and supportive friendship. Rascal and Holly are to be mentioned as well.

I give a precious thanks to my mother Shirley Cunningham who has graced my life with her love, and to the many friends who continually support my writing endeavors with encouragement, enthusiasm and respect.

Finally I want to express my appreciation for the beauty of this earth. Practicing yoga in nature has helped bring focus to this book. I wrote the book while living in a small beach house in Northern California next to the ocean and the redwoods. In between writing periods I traveled to beautiful places on the planet where I offered yoga vacations. The beauty of nature continues to inspire me. It is a healing element in my life. I am grateful for the beauty that surrounds us.

Contents

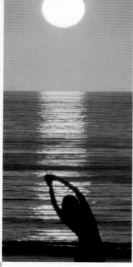

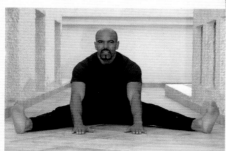

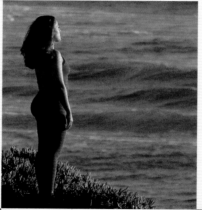

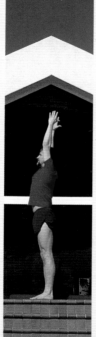

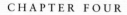

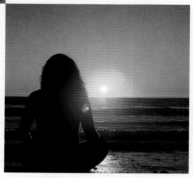

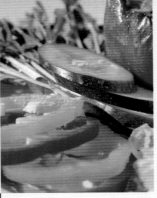

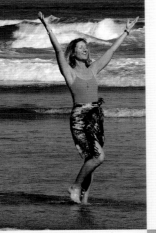

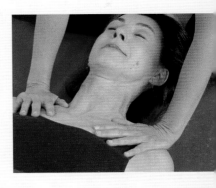

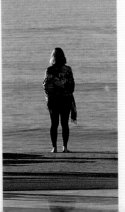

Preface

Yoga is a practice that has become quite popular in the last few years. When I was asked to write another book on this topic, I had to ask myself, "What can I offer that has not already been written?" And, of course, the answer is, "My own unique perspective and experience." I have been learning, teaching, and practicing hatha yoga for over 20 years. In particular, I have worked with people who were absolutely new to yoga and perhaps intimidated by the idea of taking a yoga class. I have worked extensively with college students, with people in 12-step recovery programs, and with people who have health challenges and physical disabilities. The practice I offer is gentle hatha yoga with an emphasis on mind and body healing.

My first book, *Stretch & Surrender: A Guide to Yoga, Health and Relaxation for People in Recovery,* was written specifically for people in 12-step programs who were recovering from alcoholism, addiction, and co-dependent compulsive behaviors. *Stretch & Surrender* was designed to offer gentle, simple, nonintimidating instruction in yoga, health, and relaxation practices. I purposely used models who did not have "perfect" body images. I stayed away from Sanskrit terms. The postures and exercises were easy to understand and follow. My goal was to encourage and support people who had not always known how to love and nurture themselves in positive healthy ways.

My vision was to empower these people with easy-to-learn positive living skills that would help them heal themselves and move toward wholeness.

After *Stretch & Surrender* was published, I discovered that people who were not involved in 12-step programs were also using and enjoying the book. Many people expressed appreciation for the simplicity and accessibility of the techniques offered. They liked the affirmations with the postures and the attitude I emphasized of self-acceptance, patience, and gentleness for healing. Thus I began to expand my teaching practice to include all people who are interested in self-growth and transformation.

This book is an outgrowth of *Stretch & Surrender.* It encompasses my basic vision of offering yoga tools for self-empowerment toward healing and wholeness. The techniques offered here teach us how to become more knowledgeable about ourselves, giving us tools to bring ourselves back into balance. Within the quiet of the body and mind lies a wealth of resources! Often the actions needed for healing are receptivity (the ability to listen and wait), respect for the subtle energies of the body, and nurturing a small awareness of improvement into a fully expressed strength. We have an inner wisdom that will guide us, if we listen.

A teacher of yoga is also always a student, which is one of the wonderful aspects of studying yoga. There is always more to learn. In my own life, different styles of yoga were attractive to me at different times. When I first learned about yoga, I had emotional healing work to do—I needed to learn to release the stress in my body, quiet my mind through meditation, and just be still. I became certified in the Ananda Yoga tradition, which teaches a gentle, inward-directed hatha style with the in-depth study and practice of meditation.

As I became more familiar with the postures, I began to explore other styles and discovered an appreciation for a more flowing and challenging yoga practice. I became certified as a teacher of White Lotus Yoga, developed by Ganga White and Tracy Rich, who taught me the flow series. I liked the challenge, the flowing pace, and the workout that made my body strong yet flexible. I remember feeling extremely healthy and full of life as a result of my daily practice. I took the training for three consecutive years. I incorporated the flow series into my classes, yet continued to teach the slow and gentle hatha yoga for my beginning students. Life was good, and I felt blessed to be teaching yoga and giving massages for a living.

Then one month after my fortieth birthday, I was in a car accident that left me with many injuries. I had torn ligaments and tendons throughout my body. I was told to limit my stretching, and certainly the pain I experienced limited my movement. I learned that soft-tissue damage does not heal quickly. It took close to a year for my body to heal. For the first time in my life, I felt old and limited by the pain I experienced. I was forced to let go of my massage practice, which had been a vital part of my income. And I began to wonder if I could still teach yoga.

With plenty of time to reflect about my life, I also deepened my exploration of how to practice yoga while limited by injuries and pain. I literally had to reinvent my yoga practice. I began with my

breathing. Daily pranayama practice helped to relax my body and calm my mind. Meditation was more challenging in the beginning because of the physical pain I experienced. I found that listening to chants was more helpful for focusing my mind.

Maintaining a positive attitude was essential. The truth is that I was depressed. The accident forced a lifestyle change that I did not welcome at the time. I was used to being very active—I enjoyed dancing, hiking, bike riding, yoga, travel, and giving massages. After the accident, I had to stop activities that I had taken for granted. If a friend invited me to go on a canoe trip, I had to inform him that I could not row. Lifting things was impossible. There were many limitations that I was forced to embrace during that time. The good news is that our bodies do heal, but it takes time— it took patience, compassion, perseverance, and staying present with my process.

Through this experience I have gained a new respect for how our bodies heal and, more important, how we can assist in that healing. A year after the accident, I attended another yoga-certification training in Integrative Yoga Therapy developed by Joseph La Page. At the training, I could not help but compare within myself the changes in my yoga practice as a result of the injuries I had endured. Although my body had healed, I was left with scar tissue that restricted the level of flexibility and openness I used to experience. Each time I compared my body to what "I used to be able to do before the accident," I was unhappy about the difference and therefore created disharmony in my mind. An important part of my own healing process has been to stop judging and comparing my level of yoga practice to what "I used to be able to do before the accident" and to appreciate where I am at now. Self-acceptance is at the heart of finding peace.

They say we teach what we need to learn. It has certainly been true in my life. I have had to learn over and over again to have compassion for myself, to be patient and accepting of where I am now while continuing to move forward. Daily yoga practice has been one of those life-enhancing tools that has made a positive difference in my life. Yoga has assisted me in my physical healing, emotional healing, mental healing, and spiritual healing. And I have witnessed the same in many of my students. The compassion of yoga is adaptive to all.

It has now been over five years since I was in the car accident and my body has regained a remarkable level of health. The same is true of my mind and spirit. I continue to practice yoga with an emphasis on healing and compassion. My yoga practice is not about doing the perfect asana; rather it is about finding inner peace. And for that, I am grateful.

With this book I invite you to slow down, reduce stress, and allow for greater relaxation and receptivity to healing. May peace be your destination and compassion your companion on this journey.

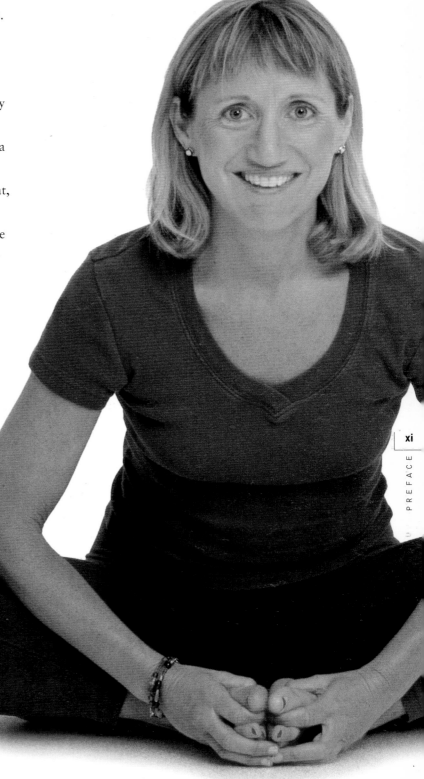

Gentle Yoga for

CHAPTER ONE

Mind and Body Healing

There are many styles of yoga practice. This book offers a slow, gentle hatha practice with emphasis on mind and body healing. Breathing practices, gentle movement, affirmations, visualizations, massage, meditation, a healthy diet, and journal writing exercises are the tools I combine to reduce stress and allow you to gain greater relaxation and receptivity to healing.

The yoga I offer is a therapeutic healing practice that assists people in finding inner peace. The theme of this practice is compassion, so that you will be extremely gentle and kind to your body and mind. Each body is unique; you don't have to be flexible or fit to practice yoga. Therefore, this practice can be used by people with physical limitations or health challenges, as well as by people who simply want to reduce stress in their lives. For example, when I teach yoga to people in wheelchairs, we work with breathing techniques, visualization, meditation, and gentle adaptive movements that work for their bodies. *Gentle Yoga* is never forceful, painful, or judgmental. Receptivity, patience, and practice are the focus of this method of healing.

Throughout this practice there is an appreciation for the breath. Students are encouraged to move *with* the breath. By allowing the body and breath to be your guide, you allow yourself to open at your own rate; you learn to surrender tensions through gentle adaptive movements rather than through force or pushing.

Compassion in our thoughts is an important factor as well. Worry and stressful thinking can affect our well-being. I think of yoga practice as a time to nourish our minds as well as our bodies. Using affirmations and visualizations for healing allows the mind to focus on the positive.

What Is Hatha Yoga?

Yoga is a system of exercise, breathing, and meditation developed thousands of years ago in India. It is the world's oldest system of personal growth—encompassing body, mind, and spirit. The goal of yoga practice is the total harmony between body, mind, and spirit in each individual and, even further, a union between the individual and the divine.

The ancient yogis understood the interrelationship among the body, mind, and spirit and the need for balance and health in all three areas as a foundation for personal spiritual awakening. The system they developed for maintaining this balance

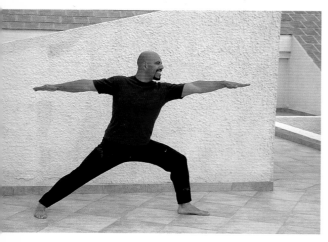

addresses body, breathing, mind, social and moral behavior, and spiritual exercises.

Hatha yoga is the branch of yoga that deals with the physical body. It is a system that combines stretching, breathing, positive thinking, relaxation, meditation, and a healthy diet to create a practical method for improving health and for developing a foundation for a deeper understanding.

Your Body Is the Vehicle That Houses Your Soul

The system of hatha yoga can be thought of as the owner's manual for a human body. Just as the owner's manual for an automobile tells you how to take care of your car, hatha yoga gives you

guidelines for taking care of your body. A car requires regular upkeep to keep it running properly. The human body is no different.

Sometimes I think that people take better care of their cars than they do of their bodies. They keep their cars clean, well fueled, lubricated, and in good working condition. Think about it. What do you do when your car gives you a warning that something is wrong? Let us say that you are driving down the road and you notice that the brake warning light on your dashboard has come on. You check to make sure that you have not left the emergency brake on. You try the brakes to make sure they still work. The chances are good that you will pull into a service station to talk to a mechanic. If he discovers that you are out of brake fluid, you gladly put more in. People want their cars to run well because they are dependent on them to go places. Your car does a lot for you, but what about your body? If you wear out your body, where are you going to live?

Our bodies are our barometers and our friends. If we learn to listen to our bodies, we will recognize when we are out of balance. Symptoms such as fatigue, neck and shoulder tightness, headache, indigestion, nervousness, or upset stomach are examples of tension signals. Fatigue is one of our bodies' first warning signs that we are out of balance in our lives. If we pay attention to this sign and allow ourselves some rest and relaxation, we can face whatever situation we are in with a clearer mind. But so often people ignore this signal. For instance, many times in my life when I felt fatigued I drank coffee so I would not notice how tired I felt.

There are many ways to mask and ignore the body's signals, but in the long run we are only doing harm to ourselves. When we ignore the small signals of the tension that is held in our bodies, we accumulate stress. Prolonged or chronic

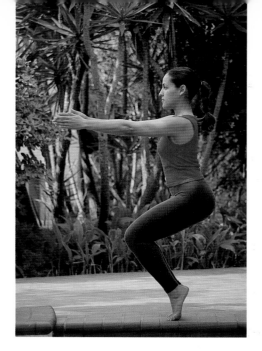

stress can result in various problems, such as migraine headaches, ulcers, backaches, high blood pressure, insomnia, breathing problems, digestive disorders, skin problems, depression, and disease.

Often it takes a severe health problem to scare people enough to reach out for help. We can only hope that by the time they get the help they need they have not done irreversible damage to their bodies. But luckily, the human body has a miraculous ability to heal. I have been amazed at how much abuse our bodies can take and, given the opportunity and proper care, still turn around and heal.

Hatha yoga offers a formula for giving our bodies the proper care they need. A healthy diet, breathing exercises, stretching, relaxation, meditation, and positive thinking are the ingredients of this formula. Practicing hatha yoga helps our bodies heal and continue to run properly. It is a practice that heals the body, quiets the mind, and gives each person a feeling of serenity.

How Does Hatha Yoga Heal the Body?

There are many physiological benefits to practicing hatha yoga. Almost immediately your body responds positively to deep breathing and stretching. You begin to relax. As you stretch your muscles, you are lengthening them. Longer muscles are more efficient and less prone to injury. The postures help you to become flexible and strong. Your internal organs are toned as well. Often, while stretching various parts of my body I think of the tin man in the *Wizard of Oz,* who needed lubrication so that he would not rust in one position. Stretching acts to lubricate the joints, muscles, ligaments, tendons, and other parts of the body. It brings movement and life energy to areas that may be tight or compressed. Greater range of motion gives you greater ease.

As you continue to practice the poses, they help flush toxins out of your body by activating and stimulating circulation, digestion, and elimination. Regular practice also helps to regulate your metabolism and the working of all the glands and organs as well as the nervous system and the mind.

The breathing exercises help to increase your lung capacity. This allows you to bring in more oxygen into your body to nourish your cells. Deep, full breathing also works to calm your emotions and lower your stress level.

The deep relaxation at the end of each yoga session quiets your mind, slows your pulse, and brings your body to a state that is receptive to healing. This allows for the total rejuvenation of your body and mind as all fatigue vanishes.

A healthy diet promotes nutritional food that contains all the necessary vitamins, minerals, amino acids, and enzymes needed to help your body heal and rebuild.

Positive thinking creates an attitude of respect and self-acceptance toward your body so that you take better care of it, as well as other aspects of yourself.

And finally, meditation allows for a feeling of tranquility and serenity that carries into all aspects of your life.

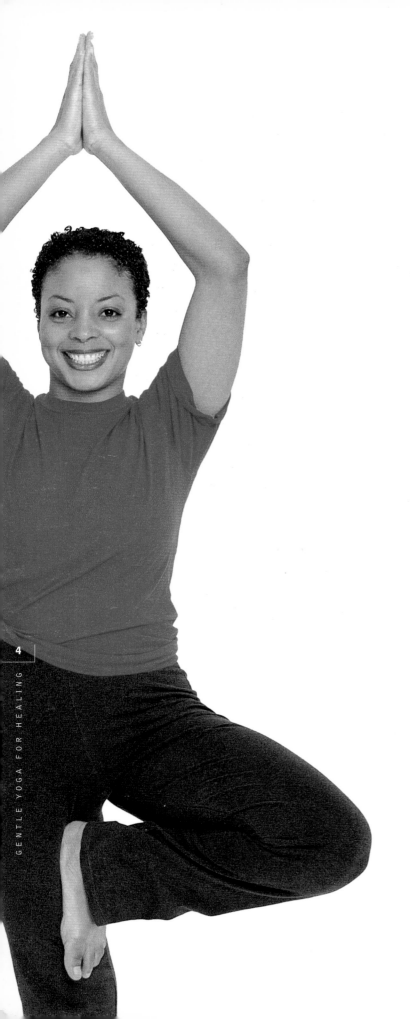

About This Book

As you read through this book you will find that each chapter introduces the various components that are a part of *Gentle Yoga for Healing*. This is a comprehensive program. All the tools offered here work together to create a healing practice.

Chapter 2 explains how positive affirmation, visualization, and journal writing are incorporated into *Gentle Yoga for Healing*. Using affirmations and visualization during yoga practice emphasizes the mind-body connection. Journal writing is another tool for becoming conscious of our innermost thoughts and feelings. I've found that writing immediately after practicing yoga is an ideal time because we are more in touch with our intuition when we are relaxed. I have developed several writing exercises, which I introduce into my yoga classes after the period of relaxation. These exercises are given throughout the book, along with visualizations.

Instruction for breathing is introduced in Chapter 3. Breathing exercises bring more energy into our bodies, calm our minds, and enhance our ability to relax. Just as the waves of the ocean continuously flow in and out, day and night, our breathing flows in and out until the day we die.

Chapter 4 gives instruction of gentle yoga postures with affirmations. 35 postures are included with specific guidelines and photos.

Gentle Yoga postures are always followed with deep relaxation described in Chapter 5. This is one of the most healing of all the practices offered. As we learn to deeply relax our bodies and minds we are more receptive to healing.

Prayer and meditation, also introduced in Chapter 5, are skills used for focusing and quieting our minds and for connecting to a spiritual presence in our lives. Spirituality has different meanings for different people. For some it is having a connection with God, the Goddess, a Guru, a Higher Power, the nature that surrounds us, or the divine mystery. The practice I offer does not dictate any one faith. Each individual's personal faith is honored and respected. The techniques offered allow the practice of prayer and meditation to enhance our lives with a feeling of unity, rather than separation. Inner peace is gained through these practices.

Eating well is a part of loving ourselves. Chapter 6 offers diet guidelines for enhancing your health and vitality. Eating a nutritious diet helps reduce stress and allows the body to repair and strengthen its natural defenses against disease. Healthy recipes are included in the chapter on diet, which are fun, and easy-to-make.

Healing from injury and illness requires special care and attention. Chapter 7 gives suggestions for supporting this process, along with a sample gentle yoga routine for people who are dealing with these challenges. The compassion of yoga is adaptive to all.

As a massage therapist I have witnessed the therapeutic value of touch for many years. With partner yoga it is easy to incorporate therapeutic neck and shoulder massage, described in Chapter 8, into your practice. Learning self-massage techniques is also very valuable. Healing touch is another tool for releasing tension in the body.

Spending time in nature is also encouraged. I often combine yoga practice with hiking in the mountains, swimming in warm oceans, meditation by a stream, or traveling to sacred power spots where the Earth's magnetic healing energy is more evident. Suggestions for connecting with the Earth's energy are included in Chapter 9, along with a section on yoga and swimming with dolphins.

The fact that yoga is a lifetime practice is emphasized in Chapter 10, which concludes the book, but not the journey of yoga.

Empowerment

This book is about nourishment, replenishment, slowing down the pace, slowing down the mind chatter, releasing stress, increasing energy, and honoring oneself through compassion and a commitment to health and wholeness. Engaging in your own healing process is self-empowering.

Gentle Yoga for Healing Mind, Body, Spirit combines these tools to create a lifestyle that enriches one's health and well-being. True wealth is health on all levels: physical, mental, emotional, and spiritual. The practices offered here focus on health and wellness within the context of spiritual growth and development. Ultimately, yoga becomes a journey to discovering one's true nature.

May all beings be well.
May all beings be free from suffering.
May all beings be happy.
May all beings live in peace.

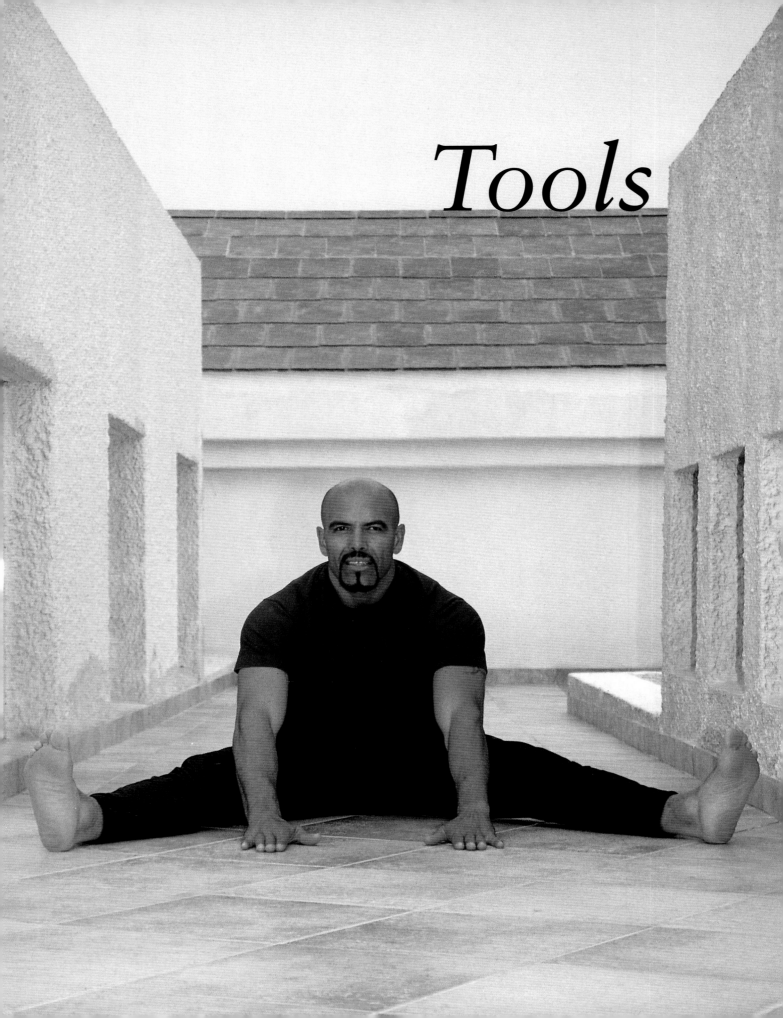

Tools

for Living

Gentle Yoga for Healing Mind, Body, Spirit works with your body and mind simultaneously by including affirmations with each yoga posture so that you use your thoughts for nurturance while stretching your body. Visualization also is used to assist you in the healing process in exercises offered in this book. Journal writing is another tool that helps to bring your thoughts and feelings, and how they affect your life, to your awareness. This chapter explains these three tools in detail.

Affirmations

In my yoga practice I have assigned a positive affirmation to each yoga posture. Say the affirmation silently to yourself while holding the pose. This combination of positive thinking with the postures is extremely powerful. You are sending an emphatic message to your own mind and emotions that recognizes the mind-body connection. Our thoughts do affect us. At the same time, the affirmations improve the quality of the pose by reminding you of the real purpose of the exercise. For instance, while doing the Camel Pose, which requires lifting up the breastbone and opening the chest as you arch back, the affirmation is "I am open and receptive to life's lessons."

Thus, the opening and healing are achieved on three levels simultaneously as I physically demonstrate, mentally affirm, and spiritually acknowledge my receptivity to my life. This integration allows inner learning to take place on a deeper level. It allows me to fully benefit from the interconnections between my physical, mental-emotional, and spiritual self.

When I first began practicing hatha yoga I remember attempting to get into a pose and thinking to myself, "I am so stiff! I am never going to be able to do this pose," and "Gosh, I need to lose weight." And sometimes my mind wandered to the various worries and challenges I had going on in my life. Even though I was helping myself physically by practicing the poses, my thoughts were counterproductive.

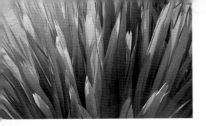

I found that making up affirmations to hold in my mind while I am holding the yoga postures was very helpful. Each affirmation is attuned to the inner feeling of the pose and helps develop self-worth. As you breathe in nurturing oxygen, use your thoughts to nurture yourself as well. Even a few concentrated minutes of a self-affirming thought can be healing. Affirmations teach us to think positively and to open our minds to loving and accepting ourselves. I like to think of my yoga practice as a time to wash away all negative thinking, all worry and fret, and to allow my mind to focus on the positive.

Positive affirmations can help reinforce a positive attitude. If you find yourself dwelling on the negative, deepen your breathing to interrupt a negative thought. Then replace it with something positive. The use of affirmations, not only in your yoga practice, but throughout your day, can make a profound difference in your inner and outer environments.

Visualization

Visualization is another tool for focusing the mind on the positive as an adjunct to healing. Visualization, or creative imagery, can be described as thought awakening the senses: hearing, sight, touch, smell, taste, and movement. Using thought to awaken your senses brings images clearly to your mind so that you experience the feelings associated with those sensations.

For instance, visualize yourself on vacation in Hawaii. Imagine the smells of tropical flowers, the sound of ocean waves, the touch of warm sand beneath your feet, the taste of fresh papaya, and

the sight of beautiful beaches. Chances are, if you have ever been to Hawaii, it will be easy to bring these sensations to your present experience. What is important about this process is that if your vacation in Hawaii was pleasurable and relaxing, then your body will respond to this visualization by physiologically becoming more relaxed. On the other hand, if you went to Hawaii and had a stressful experience, your body will respond to this visualization by becoming tense. The key to visualization is to choose images that you perceive as positive.

During yoga classes, I encourage students to use positive visualization throughout the practice. While stretching your body, visualize energy moving through your body, releasing tension and allowing for a greater openness. If there is a pose you cannot do, you can visualize yourself in that pose while focusing on your breathing. When you find an area of tension or constriction, visualize that area relaxing and opening.

This tool is particularly helpful for those people who are healing from injuries or illness. They may

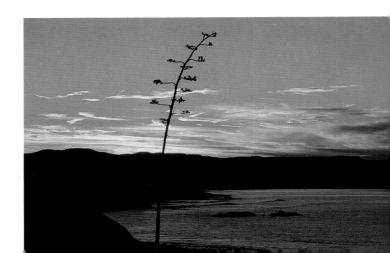

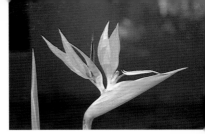

not be able to practice all the yoga postures, but they can use the time visualizing healing energy going to the injury or place of distress. I sometimes ask participants to place their hands gently on the injury or general place of illness and imagine sending healing energy from their hands into the body area that is in need of healing. Other times I simply suggest they lie down on their backs and visualize a warm healing light shining down on their body, sending healing energy to every cell in their body. With each inhalation, they can imagine healing energy, vitality, and peace entering their body; and with each exhalation they can imagine all tension and anxiety leaving their body. Using their imagination in this way is proactive at a time when sick or injured people may feel quite helpless. Visualization allows us to become engaged in our own healing process.

Visualization can be used any time you want to feel more relaxed and at peace. It can have profound effects on your mind-body experience. Take time each day to imagine yourself as a healthy person. Imagining yourself in a very beautiful, peaceful, and quiet place that you love is a simple exercise in visualization. It is like daydreaming on purpose. When using visualization, it is helpful to make it as real as you can, activating all your senses to create the inner experience. Imagine sounds, sights, smells, textures, and movements that all help to stimulate memory and emotion. The more detail you use, the better.

You will find healing visualizations throughout this book. It's also fun to write your own. With daily practice, visualization can become another tool that will enhance your health and well being.

Journal Writing

Journal writing is an invaluable tool for deepening our relationship with ourselves. Journal writing teaches self-expression and acceptance. It helps us to become more conscious of our innermost thoughts and feelings.

I have found that taking time for journal writing immediately after practicing hatha yoga and meditation is ideal because these practices enable me to experience a state of peace and receptivity: I am relaxed, I have quieted my being, and I am more in touch with my intuitive self. Personal insights flow. Divine, intuitive guidance is received. The pen records my thoughts with clarity and ease.

Journal writing is especially helpful when you are facing a challenge. Writing about your feelings gives them expression. You move the energy from inside your body through the pen to the paper. If you are feeling anxious, fearful, angry, or sad about something, just the act of writing down your feelings is helpful in gaining perspective. You become a witness to what has been written down and gain understanding about your personal process. Writing also offers validation to your thoughts and feelings as you give them a voice on paper.

I usually introduce a theme for writing at the end of yoga practice after talking students through a visualization relaxation process. As my students slowly sit up after the relaxation, they have a paper and pen next to them for their use. I ask them to not speak to one another but instead to take some time for writing. As the hand becomes occupied, the mind further quiets and revelations flow.

Relaxation visualization

Record the visualization on a tape to play back to yourself, or ask a friend to read it slowly to you. Do this after your yoga practice, during the period of relaxation. Have a notebook and pen ready for writing.

1. Lie down on your back. Place your arms along the sides of your body with palms face up. Push your shoulders down toward your feet. Allow your teeth to be slightly parted so that your jaw is relaxed. Close your eyes and deepen your breath. Take several deep breaths as you allow your body to relax.

2. Imagine that you are resting on a warm sandy beach near a beautiful ocean. The soft grainy sand underneath your body is supporting you completely. You feel your body sinking into the sand. Take some deep breaths and smell the fresh salty air. In the distance you hear the sound of the ocean waves flowing in and out, just as your breath continues to flow in and out. Allow yourself to relax even more. Above you the sky is slightly cloudy with ocean fog. Yet there are gentle sun rays of light shining through the fog, warming your body. You feel the sunlight on your face and your body becomes more and more relaxed. Breathing in and out, you are at peace.

3. When you are ready to get up, come out of the relaxation slowy. Begin by gently moving your hands and your toes. Slowly roll your body to one side and use the palms of your hands against the floor to help you sit up.

4. Find the pen and paper to begin writing.

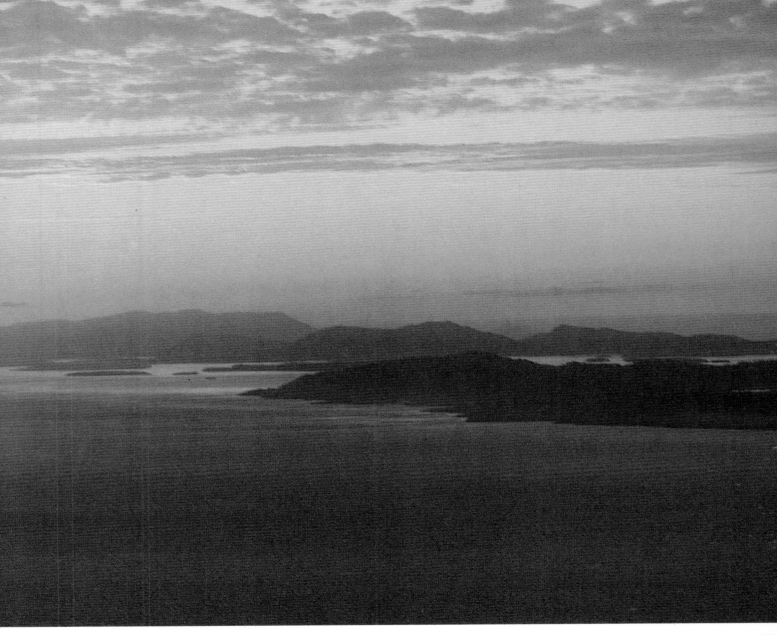

Journal writing exercise

1. Write down the answers to these questions:

   Are there any areas in your life that seem to be "foggy" right now?

   What situations or decisions are you unclear or unsure about?

   Can you find any rays of clarity shining through?

2. Describe the situation and your feelings about what is happening.

3. Notice if you gain any clarity when you put your thoughts on paper. Write about the clarity that you do have. Allow the voice of your intuition to come forth, even if it seems silly or not very rational.

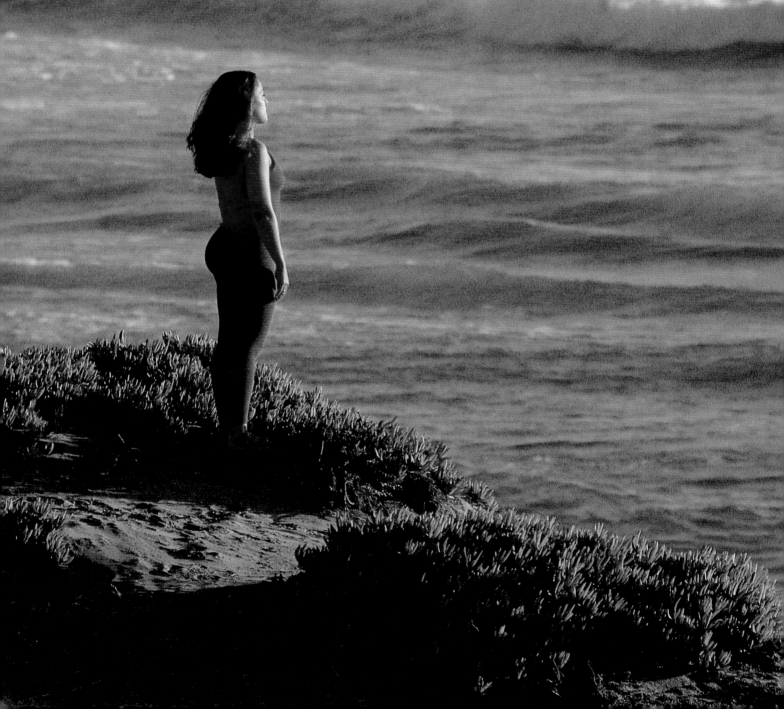

Breathing and

CHAPTER THREE

Finding Peace

Breathing is the essence of yoga. It is also the essence of our life. The Sanskrit word for breath is prana, which is also the word for energy. And that is what breath gives us—energy. Breath is our life force. As long as we breathe, we are alive. We can go for days without sleep, food, and water, but we can live for only mere minutes without breathing. Human life begins with our first breath and ends with our last. What happens in the passage between these two breaths reveals the quality of the life we have lived. If our life is filled with stress and tension our energy, health, and well-being are compromised.

Proper breathing is intrinsically linked with relaxation, with the emotions, and with the health of the body itself. When we are tense, we have a tendency to hold our breath or to take rapid and shallow breaths. When we are depressed or emotionally upset, our breathing becomes uneven. When we are frightened, we may gasp or hold our breath. When we are angry, our breathing becomes rapid and choppy.

On the other hand, when we are relaxed, our breathing becomes slow and even. The more deeply and slowly we breathe, the more we nurture and relax our entire body. Complete breathing oxygenates the blood, which in turn feeds the organ systems in the body. As you learn to breathe slowly and deeply, you will calm your mind and quiet your emotions. You cannot remain worried and upset for long if you are breathing in a calm and controlled manner. Deep breathing is a tool for getting a handle on your emotions, calming your mind, and relieving your body of tension.

If you are like most people, you probably live your life without paying attention to the way you are breathing. Unless you suffer from asthma, emphysema, or some other breathing impairment, your breathing is more or less an automatic process. Yet the breathing process lends itself easily to conscious control. With practice you can learn to breathe deeply and fully so that you get the highest benefit from each breath you take.

Diaphragmatic Breathing

One of the easiest ways to learn to breathe fully is to practice while lying down on your back. I like to practice the following diaphragmatic breathing exercise just before I go to sleep. It is especially helpful if I have a lot on my mind and am having trouble getting to sleep. As I focus my mind on my breathing, I let go of my thoughts, my body relaxes, and I drift off into the Land of Nod.

1. Lie down on your back and place your right hand on your lower abdomen. Breathe through your nose while you do this exercise.

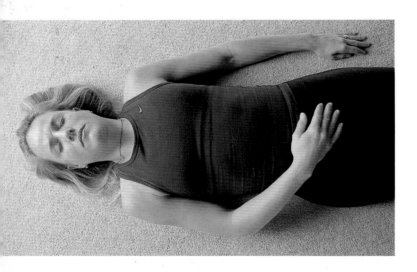

2. As you inhale slowly, think of bringing the air all the way down to the lower abdomen so that your stomach expands with the incoming air. If your hand is resting on your stomach, you will feel it rising with the incoming air.

3. As you slowly exhale, you will feel your hand lowering and your stomach hollowing with the release of air.

4. Continue breathing slowly and deeply until you have completed 10 breath cycles.

Practice this technique as often as possible so that it becomes easy for you to do.

The Complete Breath

Once you feel comfortable breathing deeply while lying on your back, you can incorporate deep breathing into your daily life. Practice the following complete breath exercise while sitting or standing, at any time during the day.

1. Begin by inhaling the air all the way down to your lower abdomen so that your stomach and lower back expand with the incoming air. Continue bringing air in so that your rib cage expands, and finalize the inhalation with an expansion of your chest so that your collarbones rise slightly. With this complete breath your entire torso is filled with oxygen, which helps nourish and relax all the muscles and cells in your body.

2. Exhale slowly in the same manner. Begin by releasing the air in your chest, then releasing the air in your rib cage, and finally emptying your abdomen so that your stomach hollows with the release of breath.

You may have noticed that there are three body parts in the complete breath. A good way to practice experiencing the breath in your body is to place your hands on each part while you are breathing.

1. Begin by placing your hands on your abdomen as you practice several complete breaths. Breathe through your nose and feel the belly expand with the inhalation, like a balloon filling up with air. As you exhale you feel the belly gently hollow.

2. Next, place your palms on the sides of your ribs with your fingers coming around to the front. Feel the ribs expanding with every inhalation and gently contracting with every exhalation. Bring the air all the way into your abdomen and continue bringing air into the rib cage, where your hands are now.

3. Finally, place your hands on your chest with your fingers resting on your collarbones. Feel the chest and collarbones gently rise as you complete the inhalation and gently fall as you begin the exhalation. The entire torso moves in rhythm with the breath, fully expanding and slowly contracting, gently and naturally.

With practice you will be able to breathe this way smoothly and continuously. As you continue to practice this breath, you will notice that the exhalation will gradually become twice as long as the inhalation. The exhalation is the letting go; most of us have stress and tension that need letting go. Inhale rich oxygen, and as you exhale let go of all stress and tension in the body. If you let all the air out completely, then the inhalation comes back naturally. Fill the torso and then take time to exhale out, enjoying the feeling of lengthening the breath and letting go. By encouraging a long, slow exhalation we are activating the parasympathetic nervous system, which allows us the feeling of relaxation.

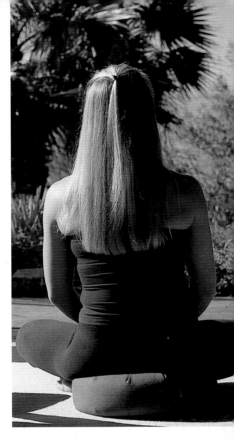

Prana (Life Force)

The Sanskrit word prana means breath, energy, and life force. The yoga perspective teaches that prana is the vital life force that pervades all of existence. This prana is evident and moves through all of life. The ocean waves move in and out; we breathe in and out; the Earth breathes and rotates—everything is energy moving.

Prana is intimately linked to the breath, which is both the major source of prana and serves as a vehicle for regulating the flow of prana throughout the body. Other important sources of prana are sunlight, water, live foods such as fresh organic vegetables, and nature. It is common to feel energized in natural environments, such as at the ocean, in the mountains, near the redwoods, by rivers, or creeks. These areas are full of prana. They have a natural life force that affect us in positive ways. I like to encourage my students to actively access prana in simple ways, such as going barefoot on the earth, swimming in the ocean, eating fresh vegetables from the garden, and, of course, taking deep full breaths of the energy that surrounds us.

Prana is something that can be experienced within the body. As we focus on our breath, we may feel a sensation of warmth moving through the body, sometimes experience a gentle coolness, and often become aware of moving energy. In fact,

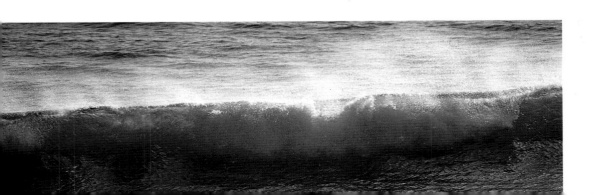

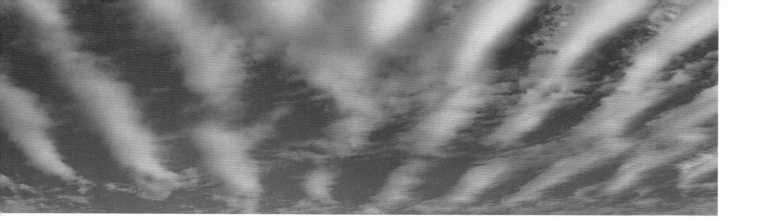

when prana flows freely through our body, we have more energy.

On the other hand, when prana is blocked, we have less energy. Tension, tightness, and contraction in the body create energy blocks that lessen the flow of energy. Yoga aids the process of removing these tensions and the underlying thought patterns that sustain tension. We then experience a greater flow of life energy and our true physical, mental, and spiritual health is enhanced.

Pranayama (Breath Control)

The science of breath control is called pranayama. (Yama means control, restrain, or channel.) Pranayama is used to channel and expand the prana, the life force. The yoga tradition teaches that we have a certain limited number of breaths in each life. As we lengthen the breath, we also lengthen our life span.

The breath is the bridge between the body and the mind. Breathing exercises help to calm the mind. Breathing can also be a great aid in energizing the mind. Shallow breathing left undetected is a signal of stress. As the body and the nervous system react to shallow breathing, more stress is produced. Our breathing is directly connected to our nervous system; because of this, people feel the positive effects of pranayama almost immediately. As we practice pranayama exercises, our breath becomes smoother, calmer, more focused, which in turn clears our energy, calms our emotions, and centers our minds.

The best part about these exercises is that they are free. All they cost is the time and energy that you take to do them. I have had many students with anxiety disorders who reported that they were able to stop their medication after adopting a regular practice of pranayama exercises. Each time they felt an anxiety attack coming, they worked with their breathing practices. What a wonderful tool at our disposal! Consciously working with the breath is calming, balancing, relaxing, and energizing.

Alternate Nostril Breathing (Nadi-Sodhana)

Alternate nostril breathing is a wonderful technique for calming and relaxing your body and mind. The Sanskrit name for this practice is nadi-sodhana, which means purification (sodhana) of the nerve currents (nadis). The nadis are metaphorical nerve channels in the energy body through which prana flows. The purpose of this breathing exercise is to counteract physical and mental tension. By regulating the breath and deepening and lengthening it, you release tension from the nadis, calm the mind, and feel relaxed.

1. Sit in a comfortable position with your spine straight. For this practice, rest your left hand comfortably in your lap.

2. Place the middle and index fingers of your right hand in the center of your forehead, between the eyebrows.

3. Gently press the side of your right nostril with your thumb, closing off the right nostril. Inhale deeply through your left nostril, feeling the coolness of your

breath travel in the upper nostril and still further up inside your head.

4. Rest your ring finger lightly on the side of your left nostril. As you press your left nostril, lift your thumb from your right nostril and exhale slowly and fully out of the right nostril, feeling the warmth of the breath as you exhale. Exhale completely.

5. Now keeping your left nostril closed with your finger, inhale deeply through the right nostril, feeling the coolness of the breath.

6. When the inhalation is complete, press your right nostril, lifting your finger from your left nostril, and exhale through your left nostril.

You have just completed one round of alternate nostril breathing: inhaling left nostril, exhaling right; inhaling right nostril, exhaling left.

7. Repeat this alternate nostril breathing pattern for five rounds, making a total of six.

8. When you have completed your last round, lower your hand and breathe naturally for a minute. Close your eyes and observe how calm you feel.

If at any time you feel discomfort, simply resume normal breathing. With practice this technique will come quite easily. In the beginning, do this practice for one minute. In time you can build up to three and then five minutes.

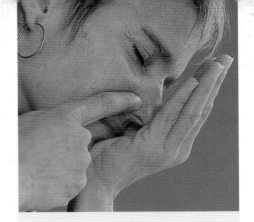

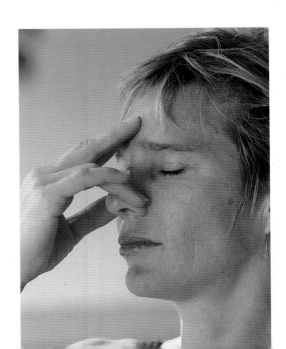

Sometimes one or both nostrils will be plugged up because of allergies or a cold. A helpful remedy is to sniff warm saltwater though each nostril, which helps loosen and clear the excess mucous and phlegm. Sprinkle a little natural sea salt into warm water (approximately 1/4 teaspoon sea salt to 1 cup warm water). Cup your hand and place some saltwater in it. Sniff some up each nostril, one at a time. As you sniff the saltwater up the right nostril, close off the left; as you sniff the saltwater up the left nostril, close off the right. If you have sinus challenges, the saltwater may sting, but it will not hurt you. Be sure to have a tissue nearby for blowing your nose. Saltwater sniff is a wonderful technique for helping to prevent sinus infections. Practiced daily, this purification exercise helps to counteract the effects of pollution, dust, and pollen.

Conscious Breathing

The simplest breathing practice is to bring conscious attention to your breathing pattern in everyday life. Notice what happens to your breathing pattern when you become busy or stressed. For instance, when you are caught in a traffic jam that is making you late, what happens to your breathing? Do you hold your breath? Does it become erratic or jagged when you are upset? When you are angry, what happens to your breathing? When you are in a hurry, how does your breathing pattern respond? Becoming aware of our breathing patterns is a revealing step toward changing our breathing so we can use our full breathing potential.

Consciously make an effort to practice deep, full, conscious breathing wherever you are. Notice that as you become calm, your breathing naturally becomes slower and steadier. And the reverse is also true—if you allow your breathing to be slower and steadier, you will become calm. It is a very empowering tool. Breathing deeply and fully helps quiet the mind and calm the emotions. If you are nervous, take deep full breaths. Remember that the deeper and slower you breathe, the more relaxed you will become. Allow your exhalations to lengthen and feel your body release its tension. This simple change can help so much in reducing stress. Full breaths provide nurturing oxygen to all the cells in your body—more oxygen, more prana, less stress. Conscious breathing is our link to greater relaxation, energy, and peace of mind.

Breathing Visualization

Close your eyes. Imagine that you are sitting on a beautiful beach, breathing in fresh ocean air. You can smell the salty quality of the air and feel the gentle ocean breeze against your skin. There is nowhere you have to go right now, and nothing you have to do but simply breathe and enjoy the beauty of the ocean. Each time you inhale, you feel peace and relaxation. Each time you exhale, you feel tension leaving your body. The ocean is relaxing and revitalizing.

As you continue to sit there on the beach, listening to the ocean waves washing in and out, your breath flows in this same pattern: breathing in, breathing out; breathing in, breathing out. Each time you inhale, you feel peace and relaxation. Each time you exhale, you feel tension leaving your body. You notice that your breathing has become slow, steady, and full. You are inhaling deep, full breaths of fresh ocean air and exhaling, releasing all tension. The calmness of the ocean is the calmness in your mind. The beauty of the sea is the beauty of your soul. Breathe and be.

Journal Writing Exercise

Think about those times in your life when you have felt at peace. Where were you? Who were you with? What were you doing or not doing? Write down what you remember of those times. Then write down a list of all the places that give you a feeling of peace. Draw a picture of a place that is peaceful for you.

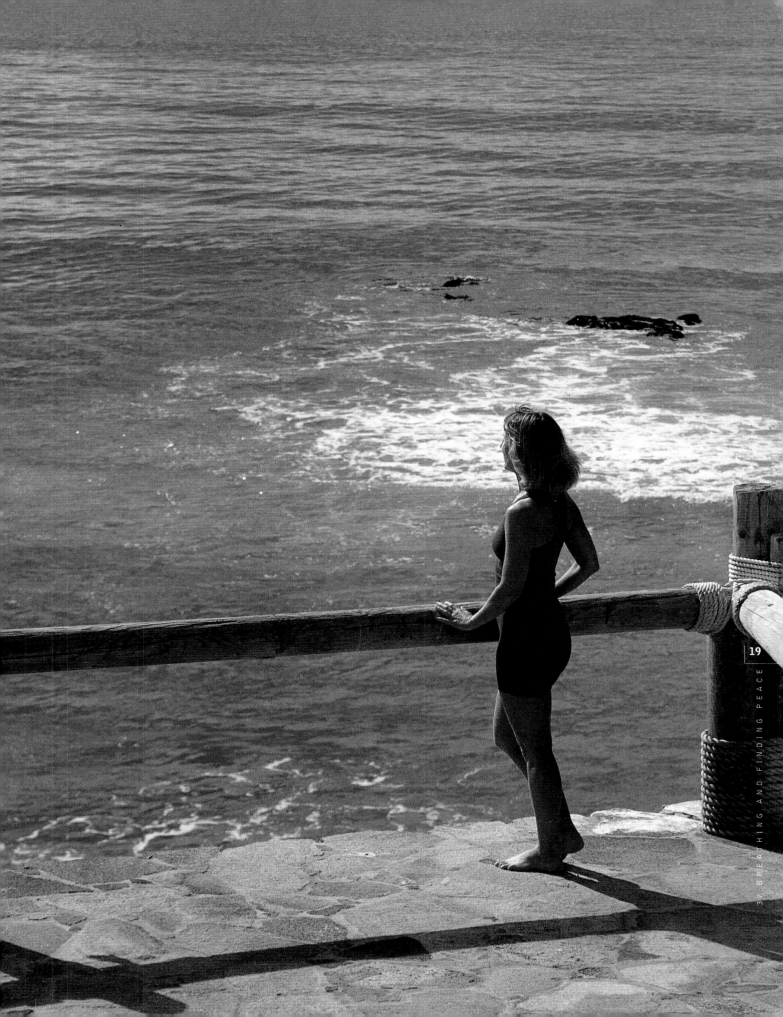

Yoga Postures

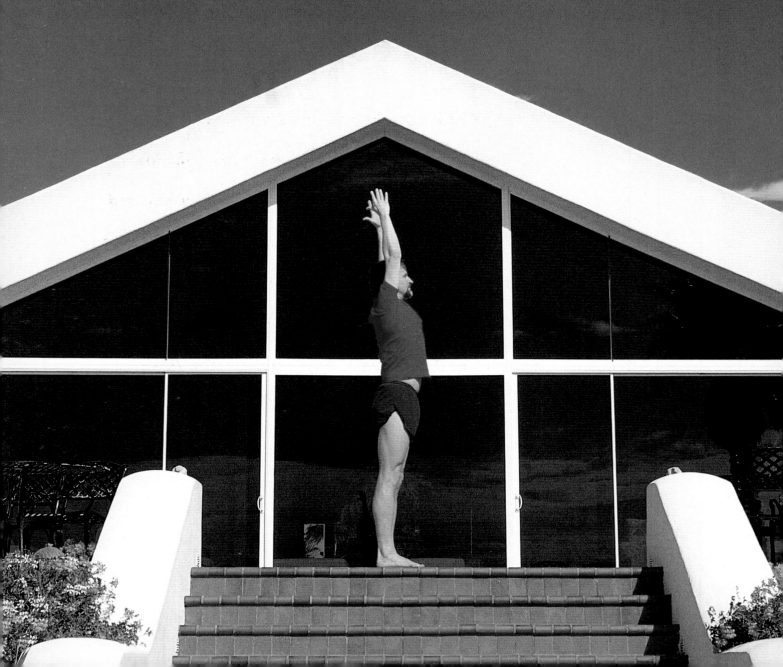

with Affirmations

In the practice of Hatha Yoga students move into specific positions or postures which are held for several moments. These positions are often referred to as asanas (pronounced ah-sah-nah)—the Sanskrit word for posture. The asanas improve the health of the body and prepare the body for sitting in meditation. There are 35 yoga postures in this chapter. Please read the entire chapter before you begin practicing the postures.

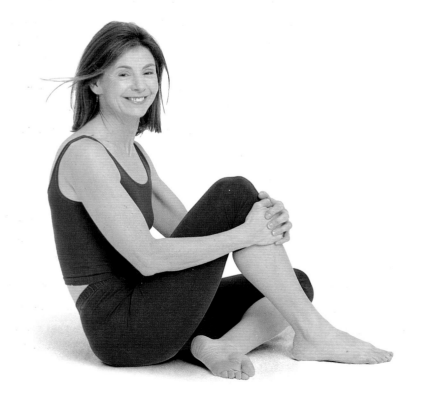

Right Attitude

There are three ingredients necessary for practicing Gentle Yoga for Healing Mind, Body, Spirit: willingness, gentleness, and patience.

Willingness

First you need to be willing to set time aside for your yoga practice. I suggest 20 minutes a day to start. The same time each day is best—consistency becomes a habit. I usually start in the morning because it starts my day with a positive feeling of well-being. Some people prefer the evening so that they can unwind from the day.

It is most important that you choose a time when you will be free from interruptions. For some people, this may sound impossible. Our busy lives leave little room for ourselves; work, children, phone calls, emails, and household responsibilities fill our waking hours. Taking time out to nurture ourselves seems like too much of a luxury. Yet those who do not take time out for self-nurturing are more likely to accumulate stress and tension, which leads to less vitality and less effectiveness. The willingness to slow down and relax is essential to our overall well-being.

With this in mind, yoga practice becomes an exercise in affirming your self-worth. Even if you start out stretching only 10 minutes a day, you are still taking little steps in learning self-care and relaxation. To help you do this I have provided suggested daily postures at the end of this chapter to allow you to start out slowly and gently, 10–20 minutes a day.

Gentleness

The second important quality for asana practice is gentleness. This requires attentive care, not only with your body but also in the way that you think. The attitude of gentleness is particularly important for those people who have injuries or health challenges. You want to be gentle with yourself, the way you would with a child.

Too many times I have heard yoga students in class criticize themselves for their lack of flexibility or for their inability to do a posture the way someone else can. When I hear this, I remind my students that yoga is not competitive—it is cooperative. As we learn to cooperate with our bodies in acceptance of where we are now, we develop self-awareness without judgment.

Judgment and criticism are the opposite of gentleness. I have often noticed that muscles behave like people. Whenever we meet someone who criticizes or judges us, we have a tendency to be less open to that person. We tighten and close our hearts for protection. On the other hand, when we meet someone who accepts us and encourages us, it is easy to be open. We feel more trusting and safe around that person. It is the same with our treatment of ourselves. If we are self-critical and judging of ourselves in our minds, the body reacts with a defensive tightening of the muscles. When we are gentle, accepting, and encouraging of ourselves, the body becomes more relaxed and open. Being gentle with our thoughts and movements assists our healing process. A gentle approach when practicing the asanas builds awareness and confidence that supports personal healing.

Patience

Patience, the third ingredient for asana practice, goes hand in hand with gentleness. You need to be patient with your body. Never strain or force a stretch. Stretch gently, going to the point of comfort and only slightly beyond that point, slowly, easily. Yoga should never hurt. The goal is not to see how far you can stretch but rather to work with your body in helping it to open and relax at its own rate of surrender. If you force a stretch beyond your body's limit, you will hurt yourself.

Learn to listen to your body. Pay attention to your body, and become aware of how your body is feeling and what messages your body is sending you. If your body feels especially tight or tense, acknowledge that feeling and move very slowly. If you move slowly, you will know when you have reached your limit. Never push past your limit; stretch slowly only to the edge of your maximum stretch. You should be able to feel the stretch, but it should not be painful.

Hold the pose at that edge and breathe slowly and deeply. Never hold your breath during a posture. People injure themselves because they move too quickly and forget to breathe. You will find that stretching becomes easier if you move slowly and breathe deeply.

Remind yourself to be patient. Do not be discouraged if you do not seem to be progressing as rapidly as you think you should be. It takes time for the body to become limber. If you are patient and you practice consistently, you will notice a positive difference in the way you feel.

Realize that some parts of your body will be stiffer than others and therefore will need special care and attention. Some people notice that one side of their body tends to be stiffer than the other. Use caution when stretching the stiff side, but always maintain a pose for the same amount of time on each side. If there is any discomfort or pain, either while holding a position or afterward, you are working too hard. Ease up and, again, be patient. Healing is a gradual process.

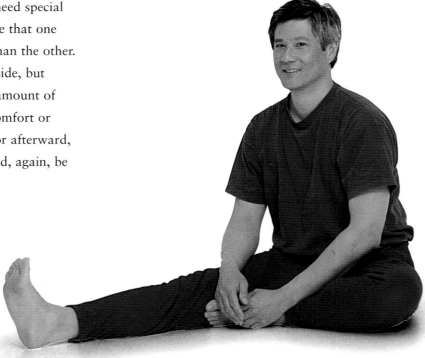

Getting Started

For the first month, follow the daily schedule guidelines at the end of this chapter. You will be adding one to three new poses each day, until you have mastered the basics of all 35 asanas.

Before you begin, read the directions for doing the poses carefully. Study the photographs. Move into the postures slowly; find a position you can comfortably hold for a minute or two. Say the affirmation listed beside the pose three times softly or silently to yourself while holding the pose. Remember to breathe deeply and fully and to coordinate your breathing with your movements. The asana instructions will guide you with your breathing. The general rule for breathing is: Breathe in whenever the body expands, opens, or reaches outward; breathe out whenever it contracts, closes, or folds. Remember to breathe through your nose.

Give attentive care to your body and breath as you practice. Do not strain; move gently and comfortably in and out of the poses. If you experience any pain as you do a pose, stop and rest; then consider how you might modify the pose for you. Your breathing will tell you if you are working too hard—if you find you cannot keep a steady deep, full breathing pattern, you need to release your effort a little. All your movements should be slow and deliberate; come out of each pose slowly. Rest for one or two long deep breaths before moving on to the next pose.

Do not neglect the deep relaxation period that follows the poses. Because it is often easier to relax when listening to instructions, you might want to record one of the relaxation scripts in Chapter 4. You can also order the relaxation CD that I have produced; information for ordering CD is listed at the back of this book on page 138. This 30-minute CD includes three visualization-relaxation scripts designed to be played at the end of yoga class or any time you need 10 minutes of guided relaxation.

And finally, for your comfort, practice hatha yoga on an empty stomach, at least one and one-half hours after your last meal, and wear loose comfortable clothing.

The Postures

1) STANDING MOUNTAIN—STRAIGHT STANDING POSTURE

The first impression we get of people is from the way they stand or walk. When people stand straight and walk with their heads high, they appear to be confident, open, and energetic. When people are hunched over, their energy is directed downward and they appear to be unsure of themselves or not as happy as they could be.

One of the first things I realized when I started practicing hatha yoga is that I had a tendency to hunch my shoulders slightly forward, which made my chest cave in rather than allowing my chest to be open and expanded. It was as if I were subconsciously trying to protect my heart and keep it from being exposed because I had been hurt so often in my life. Changing this habit took a conscious effort on my part, but in time I developed a new stance, which became a symbol of my willingness to face life's challenges with an open heart.

Practice the following straight standing posture often, especially in your daily life when you are standing in lines or standing around with others in conversation.

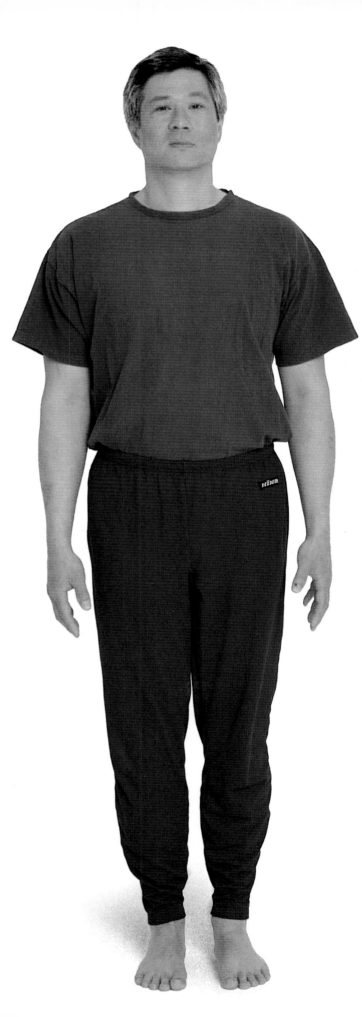

1. Begin by standing with your feet parallel.

2. Rock your weight gently back and forth until you distribute your weight equally through both your feet. Do not lock your knees.

3. Tuck your tailbone downward toward the floor.

4. Gently roll your shoulders up and back to lift and separate the rib cage.

5. Then relax your shoulders downward.

6. Let your arms relax by your sides. Your breastbone is lifted up. Your chest is open and relaxed. The back of your neck is light, feeling as though the crown of your head is lifted up toward the sky. Focus your thoughts on the affirmation.

I face life's challenges with an open heart.

7. Take several deep breaths.

Benefits

Standing Mountain pose increases awareness of body alignment and promotes good standing posture.

2) WARM UP—THE COMPLETE BREATH WITH STRETCHING

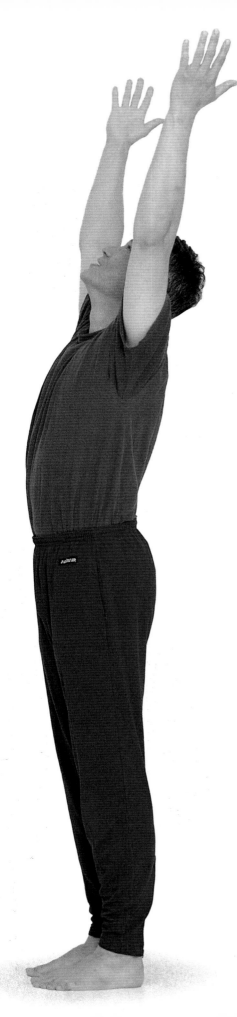

1. Begin in Standing Mountain (straight standing) posture.

2. Inhale into your abdomen as you raise your arms above your head, stretching up. Say the first affirmation.

I am filled with energy, vitality, and joy.

3. Exhale bending at the waist, folding forward as you lower your hands down toward the floor in front of you. Let your head hang freely with your neck relaxed. Allow your knees to bend slightly. Exhale all tensions, all worries, all anxiety. Say the second affirmation.

I let go of all tension, all worries, all anxiety.

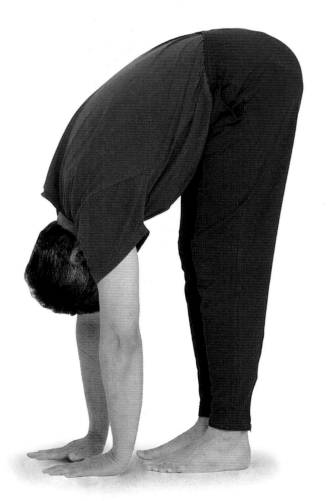

4. Inhale, rolling your spine back up, raising your arms above your head, breathing in energy, vitality, and joy. Focus your thoughts on the first affirmation.

5. Exhale and fold back down, letting go of all tension, all worries, all doubts. Focus your thoughts on the second affirmation.

6. Continue breathing in, stretching up and then breathing out, folding down. Do this five to six times. Focus your thoughts on the affirmations as you do each part.

7. With the last exhalation, remain standing while lowering your arms to your sides.

Modification

If you have a weak lower back, be sure to bend your knees as you roll back up.

Benefits

This Warm-Up exercise releases tension in the back and neck and increases energy with breath and movement. It promotes spinal flexibility and stretches the backs of the legs.

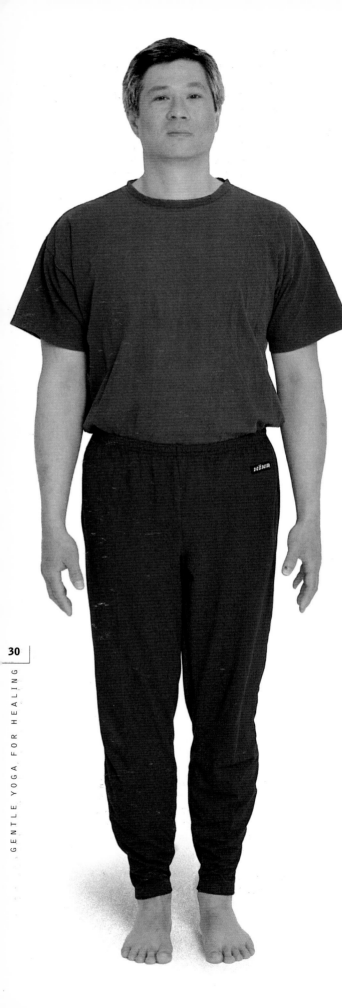

3) STANDING FORWARD BEND

1. Stand with your feet together or slightly parted, your feet pressing down into the earth. Take a deep breath. Say the first affirmation.

I breathe in energy from the Earth.

Benefits

Standing Forward Bend stretches the backs of the legs. It helps release tension from the neck and spine. Because the head drops below the heart, it is also a resting pose for the heart.

2. Exhale and fold your body forward. Allow your hands and arms to hang down toward the floor.

3. Place your hands behind your calves or ankles. If your hands are able to reach the floor, then place them outside your feet with palms pressing into the floor.

4. Draw your head down and in toward your knees. Let your neck and head relax, hanging in alignment with your spine. Let your arms hang loosely from your shoulders.

5. Hold this position as you take several breaths. Focus on the movement of your belly as you breathe.

6. Each time you exhale, feel the stretch in the back of your legs as you drop further forward. Gravity is assisting you in this stretch. Focus your thoughts on the second affirmation.

I relax my spine as I exhale.

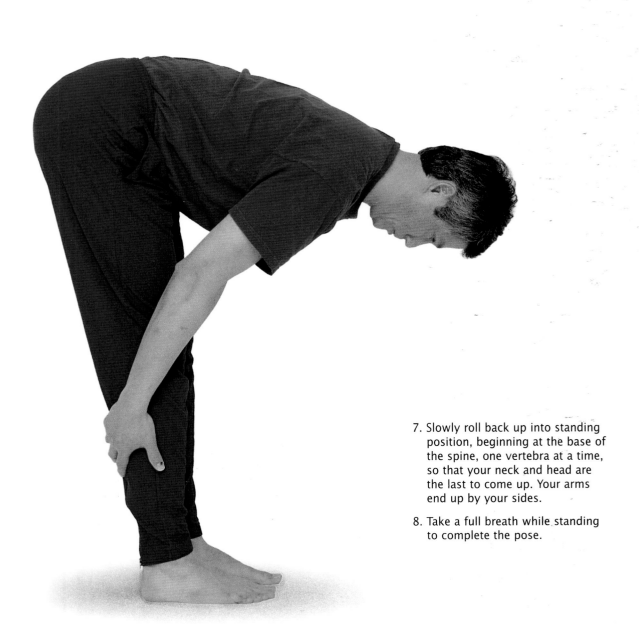

7. Slowly roll back up into standing position, beginning at the base of the spine, one vertebra at a time, so that your neck and head are the last to come up. Your arms end up by your sides.

8. Take a full breath while standing to complete the pose.

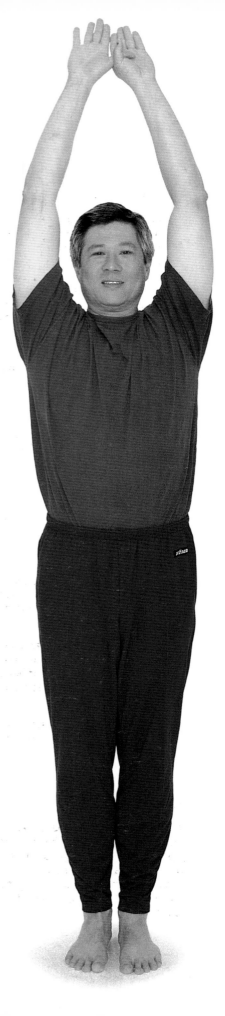

4) HALF-MOON POSE—SIDE STRETCH

1. Stand with your feet together, your weight equally distributed on both feet, your arms at your sides.

2. Stretch your hands upward, joining them above your head.

3. Inhale, lifting up onto your toes as you reach up.

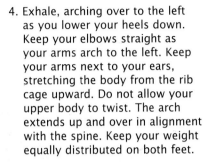

4. Exhale, arching over to the left as you lower your heels down. Keep your elbows straight as your arms arch to the left. Keep your arms next to your ears, stretching the body from the rib cage upward. Do not allow your upper body to twist. The arch extends up and over in alignment with the spine. Keep your weight equally distributed on both feet.

5. Hold the pose while breathing and feel the stretch on your right side. Focus your thoughts on the affirmation.

Strength and courage flow through me.

6. Repeat the pose arching to the right, feeling the stretch on your left side. Focus your thoughts on the affirmation.

7. Inhale up onto your toes as you stretch your hands up above your head. Exhale lowering your heels and releasing your arms to your sides.

8. Take a full breath while standing with your arms at your sides to complete the pose.

Benefits

Half-Moon Pose strengthens and relaxes the muscles on the sides of your torso. It stretches and tones the muscles along your spine, increasing circulation to the organs. It also strengthens the arches of your feet.

5) ANGLE POSE

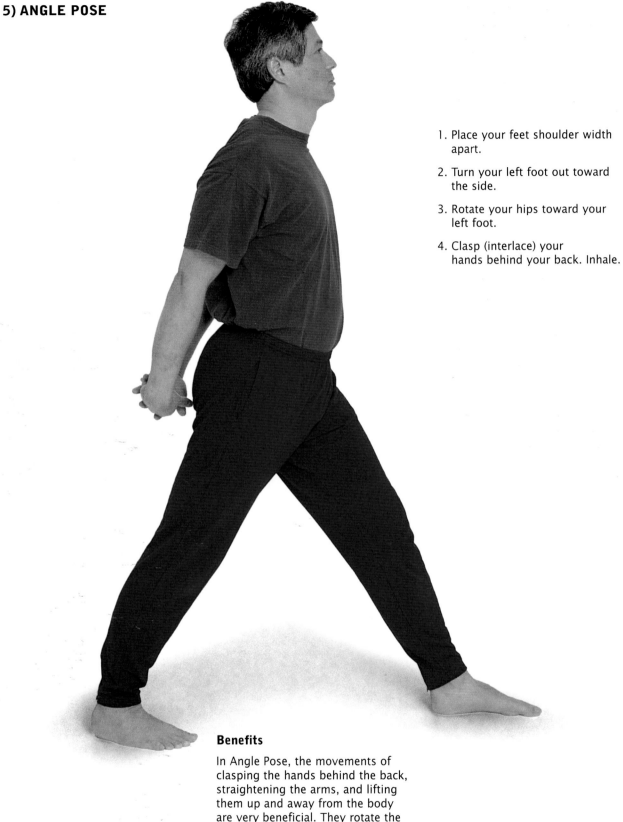

1. Place your feet shoulder width apart.

2. Turn your left foot out toward the side.

3. Rotate your hips toward your left foot.

4. Clasp (interlace) your hands behind your back. Inhale.

Benefits

In Angle Pose, the movements of clasping the hands behind the back, straightening the arms, and lifting them up and away from the body are very beneficial. They rotate the shoulders and limber up the shoulder joints, upper back muscles, and lumbar vertebrae. They also expand and stretch the rib cage and lungs, which allows fresh blood and energy into the nerves and tissues of the lungs, chest, and heart.

5. As you exhale, bend at the waist and lower your chest toward your left knee while raising your clasped hands up toward the sky.

6. Breathe as you hold the pose. Focus your thoughts on the affirmation.

I forgive myself and my burdens are lifted.

7. Inhale as you rise back up.

8. Exhale, releasing your hands and facing forward.

9. Repeat the pose on the opposite side, turning your right foot out and bending toward your right knee. Focus your thoughts on the affirmation.

10. Inhale as you rise back up. Exhale, releasing your hands and facing forward.

Modifications

You can also experiment with lifting your clasped hands only slightly or holding onto your elbows (as shown in photo).

6) TRIANGLE POSE

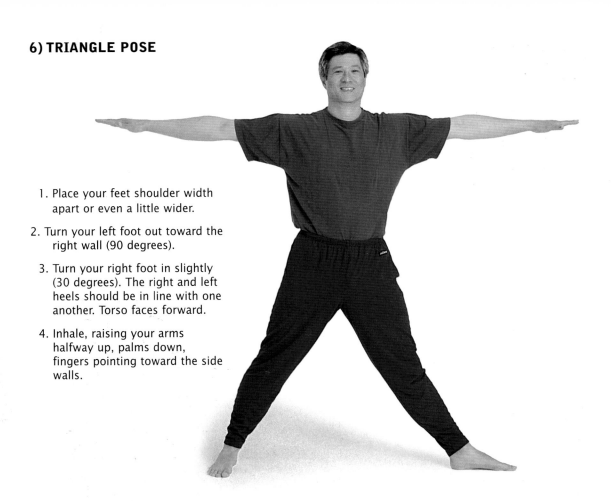

1. Place your feet shoulder width apart or even a little wider.

2. Turn your left foot out toward the right wall (90 degrees).

3. Turn your right foot in slightly (30 degrees). The right and left heels should be in line with one another. Torso faces forward.

4. Inhale, raising your arms halfway up, palms down, fingers pointing toward the side walls.

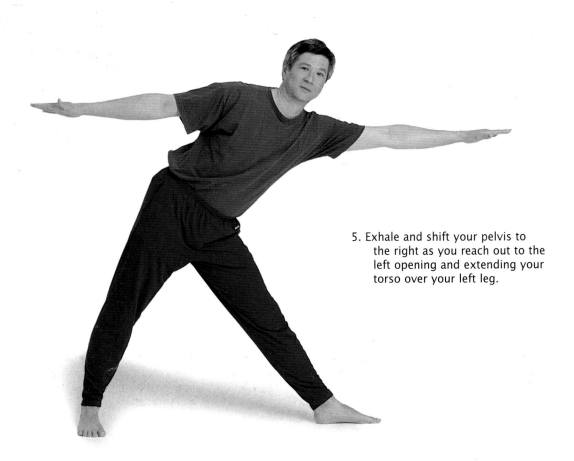

5. Exhale and shift your pelvis to the right as you reach out to the left opening and extending your torso over your left leg.

6. Lower your left hand down to your left thigh or calf while raising your right hand to point toward the sky.

7. Your right arm is now stretched upward in line with the shoulder, the palm facing forward. Turn your head to look at your right hand as you hold the pose, breathing. Focus your thoughts on the affirmation.

I am filled with acceptance and love.

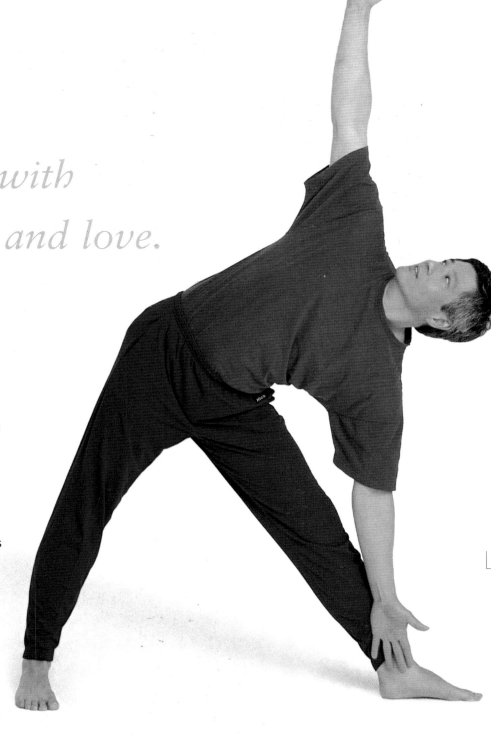

8. Inhale as you lift back up slowly, facing forward.

9. Turn your feet back to face forward.

10. Exhale as you lower your arms to your sides.

11. Repeat the pose on the opposite side.

Benefits

Triangle pose stretches the hamstrings and lateral muscles of the spine and stimulates the kidneys and adrenals.

37

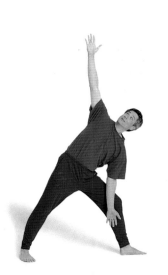

Modifications

- If your hamstrings are tight, keep the knee of your leading leg slightly bent while in the pose.

- If you have a sensitive neck look forward rather than turning your neck to look at your upper hand while in the pose.

7) THE SQUAT

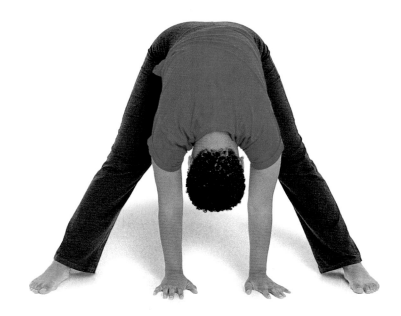

Preparing for the Squat

1. Place your feet shoulder width apart.

2. Bending down at the waist, reach down and place your hands on the floor between your feet.

3. Relax your head and neck and breathe.

The Squat

4. Inhale.

5. As you exhale, bend your knees and lower your body down completely into a squat. Your feet should be flat on the floor.

6. Bring your palms together in prayer position in front of your chest as you hold the pose, breathing. Focus your thoughts on the affirmation.

I am relaxed and centered.

Coming out of the Squat

7. Press your hands on the floor in front of you.

8. Inhale as you straighten your legs, raising your buttocks.

9. Exhale as you roll your upper torso up slowly, one vertebra at a time.

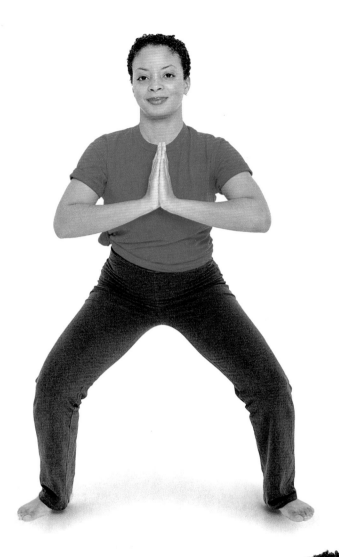

Modifications

- With practice you will be able to go into the squat from a standing position (without bending forward first).

- If you have problems with your knees or hips, proceed cautiously. Go only as far as you can without straining. Gently work within your limits. Come halfway down and hold there for several breaths. You may have problems squatting when your knees are stiff. (Yet this pose is quite natural for human beings; it is a common way to sit in many cultures.)

- At first, your feet may turn out and your heels may lift. If you cannot bring your heels flat on the ground, try widening your stance.

Benefits

The squat stretches the calf and thigh muscles and develops balance. It also helps with digestion and elimination. In the squat, the thighs press against the colon, which in turn stimulates the bowel function, stimulating the peristaltic movement of materials through the digestive tract. This pose is especially helpful if you suffer from constipation. It is also helpful for relieving lower-back discomfort from menstruation.

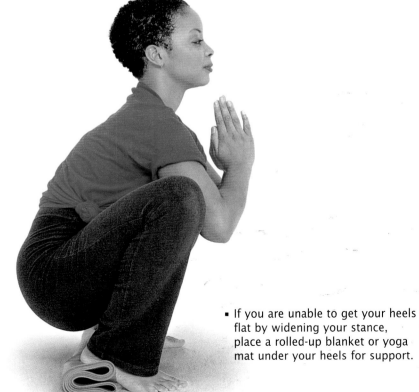

- If you are unable to get your heels flat by widening your stance, place a rolled-up blanket or yoga mat under your heels for support.

8) THE WARRIOR

1. Begin by placing your feet wide apart, as far as is comfortably possible. Your arms should be at your sides.

2. Turn your right foot out toward the right wall. Turn your left foot in slightly.

3. Inhale, raising your arms up and out to the sides until they are at shoulder level with your palms facing down and your finger pointing to the side walls.

4. Exhale, bending the right knee so that the knee is directly over your ankle, creating a right angle with your right leg. Keep your torso straight with your spine lifting upward.

5. Look toward your right hand while holding the pose and breathing. Focus your thoughts on the affirmation.

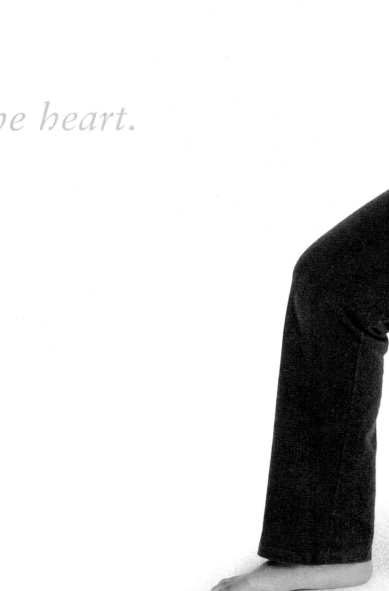

I am a warrior of the heart.

6. Exhale, releasing your arms, releasing your knee and facing forward.

7. Do the pose again on the opposite side.

Benefits

The Warrior pose gives the feeling of strength and firmness as it tones the arms and legs.

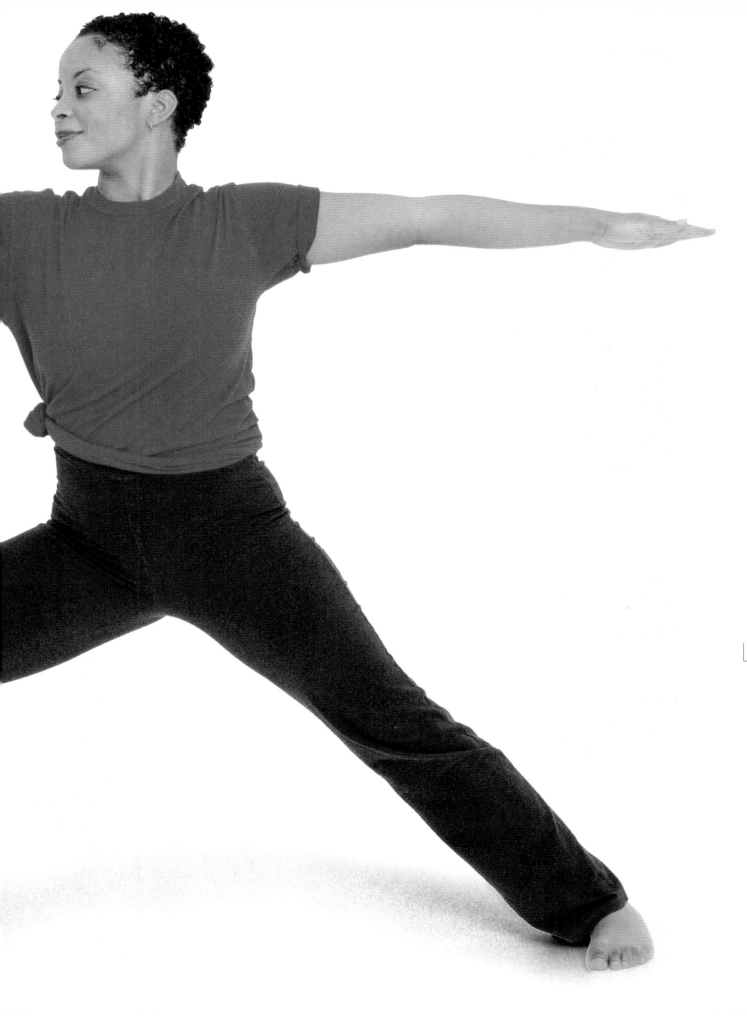

9) THE CHAIR

This is a strengthening pose. There are two phases to the pose. During both phases, you hold your arms out in front of you. You may get tired of holding them up, but remember that you are strengthening them and your thighs as well.

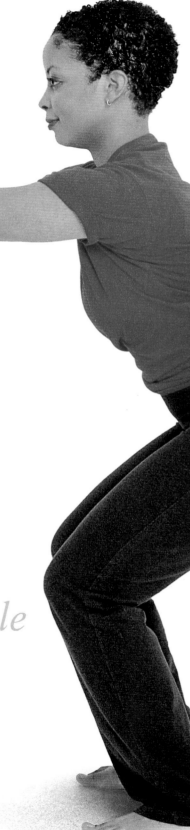

Phase 1

1. Begin with your feet slightly parted, not quite shoulder width apart.

2. Extend your arms out forward at shoulder level.

3. Inhale.

4. As you exhale, bend your knees and sit down as if you are sitting in an imaginary chair. Your knees should be directly over your feet, not pointed inward. You are sitting in midair, using your thigh muscles to keep you there. Keep your arms extended forward.

5. Remember to breathe as you hold the pose. Focus your thoughts on the affirmation.

My body is the vehicle that houses my soul.

6. Inhale, straightening your legs. Do not drop your arms. Exhale.

Caution: If you have "problem knees" or find this pose too difficult you can skip this asana or do the modification below. As you develop strength in your leg muscles it will become easier to do. Do not overdo this.

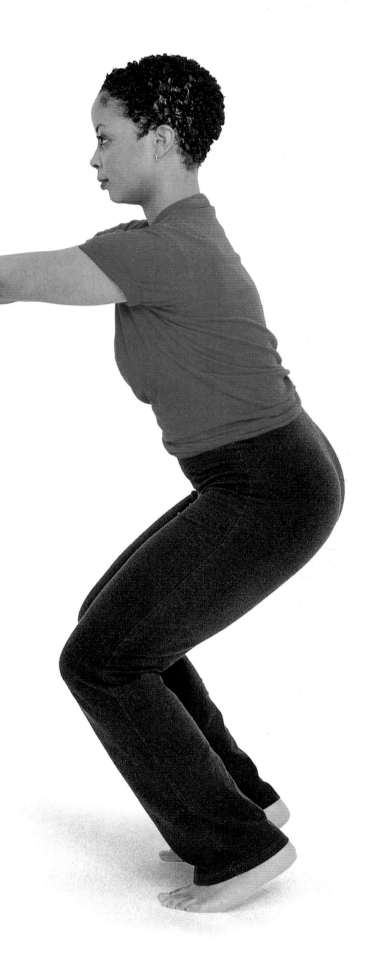

Phase 2

7. Inhale, coming up on your toes. Do not drop your arms.

8. As you exhale, sit down again into an imaginary chair, remaining on your toes. Remember to keep your knees directly over your feet. Your arms are still extended forward.

10. Breathe. Focus your thoughts on the affirmation.

11. Inhale, straightening your legs and standing up.

12. Lower your arms to your sides.

Modification

If you have knee problems then remain standing and do the arm part of the posture only, while focusing your thoughts on the affirmation.

Benefits

The Chair strengthens and tones the arms and legs. It also helps improve balance.

10) THE TREE

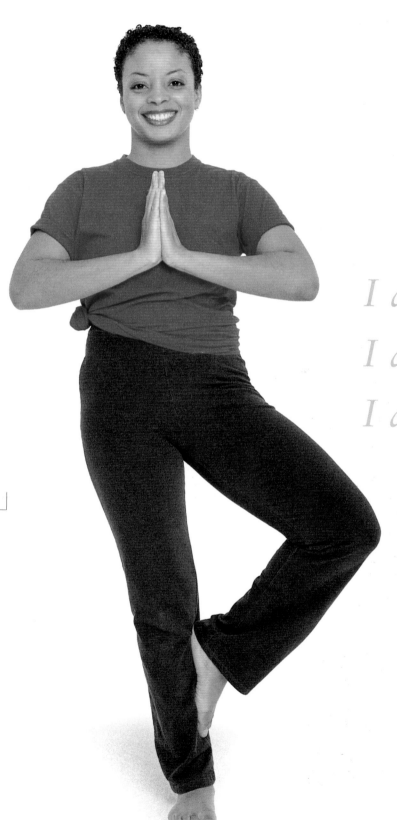

1. Begin by placing your weight on your right foot. Visualize roots growing from the bottom of your right foot going deep into the earth.

2. Focus on a stationary point in front of you.

3. Place your left foot on your left calf or thigh.

4. Inhale and place your hands in prayer position at your heart or raise them up above your head, reaching for the sky. Focus your thoughts on the affirmation.

I am calm.

I am balanced.

I am rooted in faith.

5. Exhale, releasing your arms and your foot.

6. Repeat the pose on the opposite foot.

Benefits

The Tree helps develop concentration, balance, and poise.

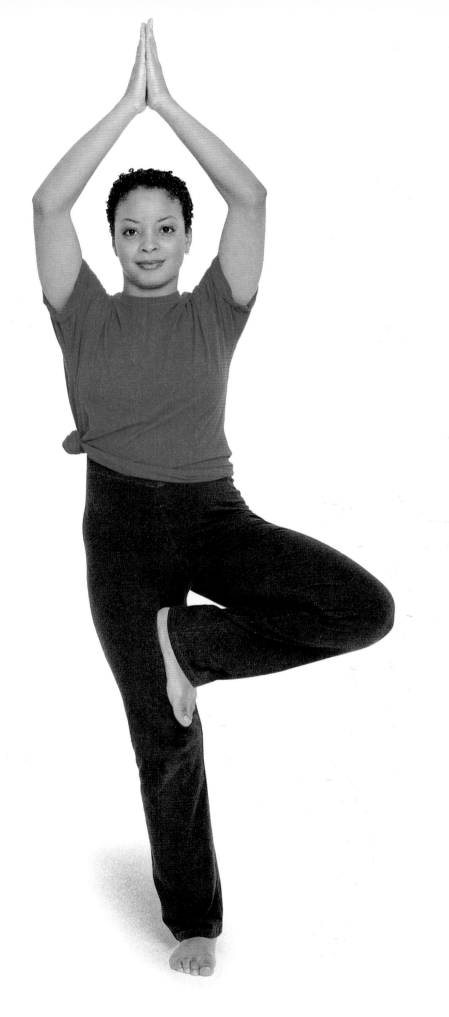

45

4/ YOGA POSTURES WITH AFFIRMATIONS

11) THE SITTING MOUNTAIN

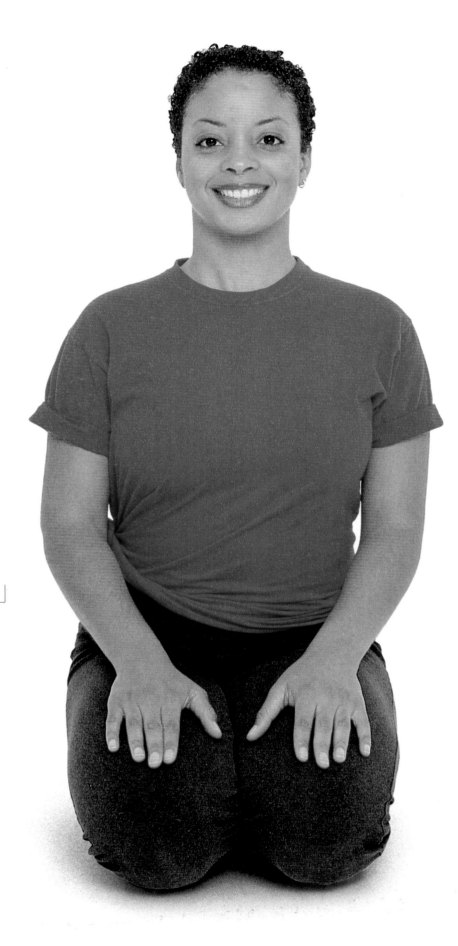

This is one of the easiest ways to sit so that your spine remains straight rather than hunched over.

1. Kneel on the floor, your knees pointed forward and your feet stretched behind you.

2. Now sit back on your heels, so that your back is upright. Relax your shoulders. Your chest should be open and relaxed. You are firmly planted like a mountain, energy going up your spine, feeling strong and calm.

3. Take deep slow breaths. Focus your thoughts on the affirmation.

Serenity comes when I surrender.

Benefits

The Sitting Mountain is a meditative pose that flushes blood from the legs as it stretches the hips, knees, and ankle joints.

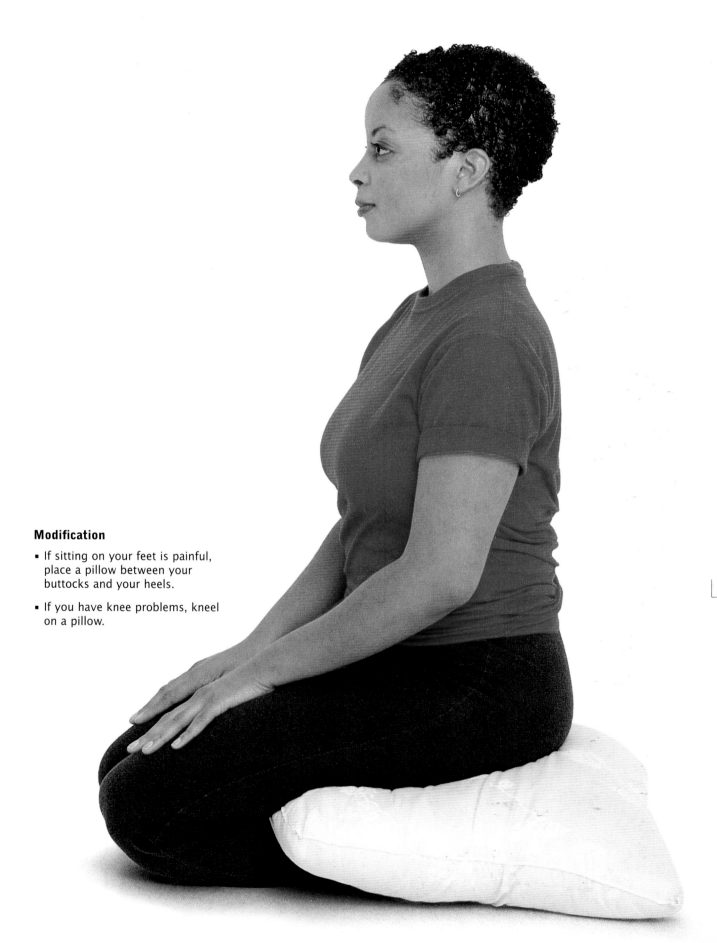

Modification

- If sitting on your feet is painful, place a pillow between your buttocks and your heels.

- If you have knee problems, kneel on a pillow.

12) CHILD'S POSE

1. Begin in Sitting Mountain pose, sitting on your feet with your toes touching and your heels separated.

2. Inhale.

3. As you exhale, gently lower your head to the floor in front of your knees.

4. Place your hands, palms up, next to your feet. Completely relax your neck and shoulders.

5. Hold this position while breathing for as long as you are comfortable. Focus your thoughts on the affirmation.

I rest in trust and patience.

6. Inhale, coming back to Sitting Mountain pose.

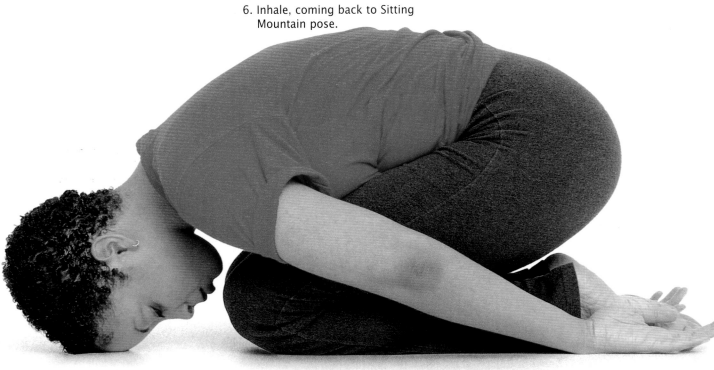

Benefits

Child's Pose allows the blood to flow to the neck and head. This pose releases tension in the shoulders and spine. It gently allows blood flow to the brain, relieving mental fatigue.

Modification

- If you have extra weight in your belly, widen your knees (slightly wider than your hips) and then lower down into the pose. Allow the head to rest on a folded blanket or pillow if that is more comfortable. You can also place a pillow between the buttocks and the legs, or begin the pose in sitting mountain with a pillow between your buttocks and your heels as shown on page 47.

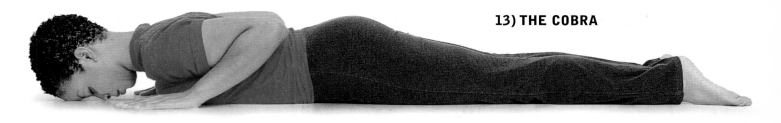

13) THE COBRA

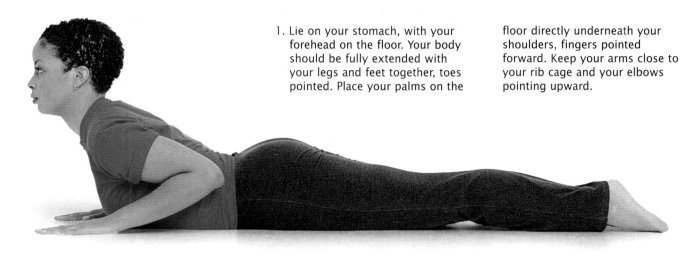

1. Lie on your stomach, with your forehead on the floor. Your body should be fully extended with your legs and feet together, toes pointed. Place your palms on the floor directly underneath your shoulders, fingers pointed forward. Keep your arms close to your rib cage and your elbows pointing upward.

2. Inhale and raise your head slowly upward. Raise your chest slightly off the floor without putting pressure on your hands. Use your upper back to hold the pose. Your hands are used for support only. Hold here for five seconds, breathing.

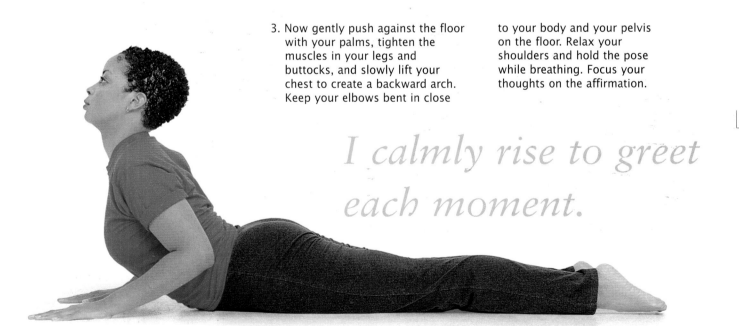

3. Now gently push against the floor with your palms, tighten the muscles in your legs and buttocks, and slowly lift your chest to create a backward arch. Keep your elbows bent in close to your body and your pelvis on the floor. Relax your shoulders and hold the pose while breathing. Focus your thoughts on the affirmation.

I calmly rise to greet each moment.

Benefits

The Cobra strengthens the upper back and vertebrae of the spine. It expands the rib cage and increases the capacity of the lungs.

4. Exhale and slowly lower your chest and forehead to the floor. Turn your cheek to the side. Place your arms down alongside your body and rest.

14) LYING-DOWN BOAT

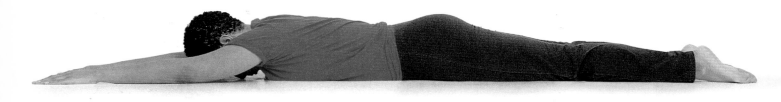

1. Lie on your stomach with your forehead on the floor.

2. Extend your arms forward, resting them on the floor. Your feet and legs should be close together and relaxed.

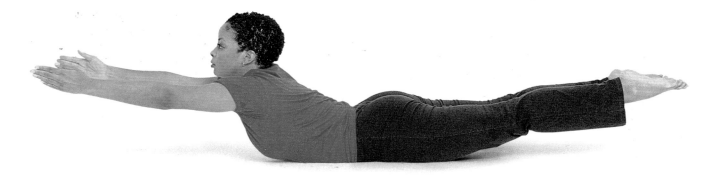

3. Inhaling, raise your arms and legs off the floor, arching up until only your stomach remains on the floor.

4. Tighten your buttocks and hold the pose—just for a moment at first, and gradually over time for up to three breaths. Focus your thoughts on the affirmation.

I reach out to others when I need help.

5. Exhale, lower your body, and relax.

Benefits

Lying-Down Boat helps to strengthen the lower back.

15) THE CAT

This pose alternates between swayback and humpback.

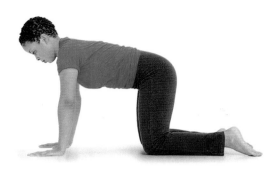

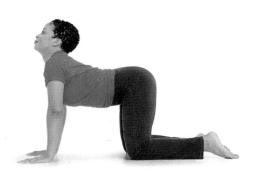

1. Kneel on all fours with your arms straight and your back parallel to the floor.

2. As you inhale, lift your head and allow your waist to lower into swayback. Hold this position for three seconds. Focus your thoughts on the affirmation.

3. As you exhale, hunch your back and let your head relax down. Hold this position for three seconds. Focus your thoughts on the affirmation.

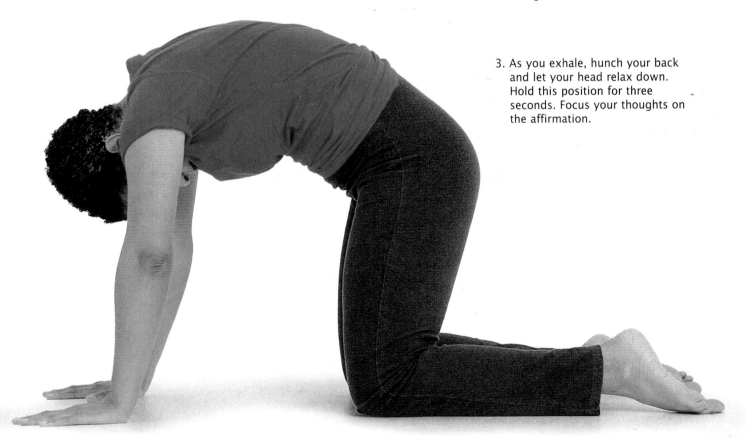

I have the option to change my attitude.

Benefits

The Cat helps stretch and strengthen the spine.

16) BACKWARD BEND

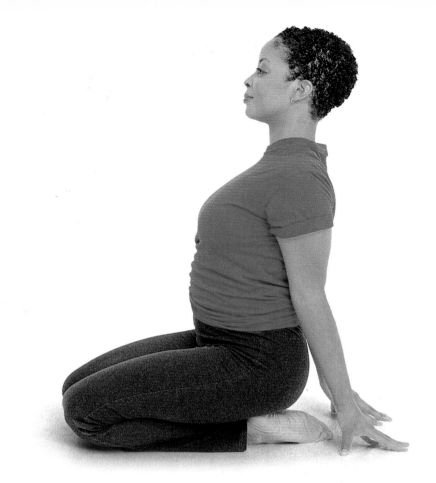

1. Start in Sitting Mountain pose, sitting on your heels, with the tops of your feet resting on the floor and your knees together in front of you.

2. Relax your shoulders and lift your chest.

3. Place your hands beside you, palms face down, fingers pointed back.

4. Little by little, walk your hands back until you reach a comfortable position where you are leaning back on your arms.

5. Relax your head and neck as you lift your chest and ribs toward the ceiling to create an arch.

6. Remain seated on your heels and breathe as you hold the pose. Focus your thoughts on the affirmation.

Modification

- Place a pillow under your buttocks before you move into the pose, if that is more comfortable.

I lean on God for guidance.

7. Release the pose by slowly shifting your chest and ribs forward, while raising your head until your chin touches your chest. Walk your hands forward to a sitting position.

Benefits

Backward Bend promotes elasticity in the spine. It stretches and lengthens the muscles across the chest. It also tones the neck and throat.

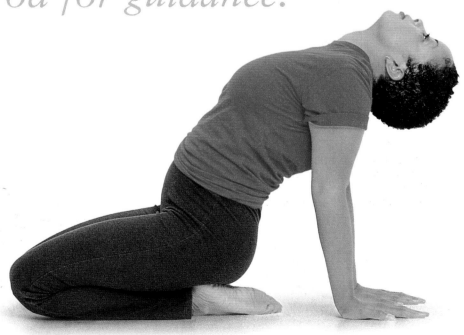

17) THE CAMEL (PREPARATION)

1. Kneel, sitting on your heels with your spine straight.

2. Inhale and rise upward so that you are still on your knees, with your body erect over your knees.

3. Separate your knees slightly.

4. Place your hands on your lower back and arch your spine, lifting your sternum and expanding your chest. Focus your thoughts on the affirmation.

I am open and receptive to life's lessons.

5. Slowly release your hands and lift back up to an erect kneeling position. Lower your body. Fold forward into the Child's Pose.

Benefits

The Camel Preparation pose expands the chest and stretches the shoulders. It is helpful for people who tend to round their shoulders.

18) DOWNWARD-FACING DOG

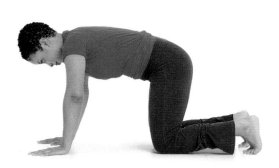

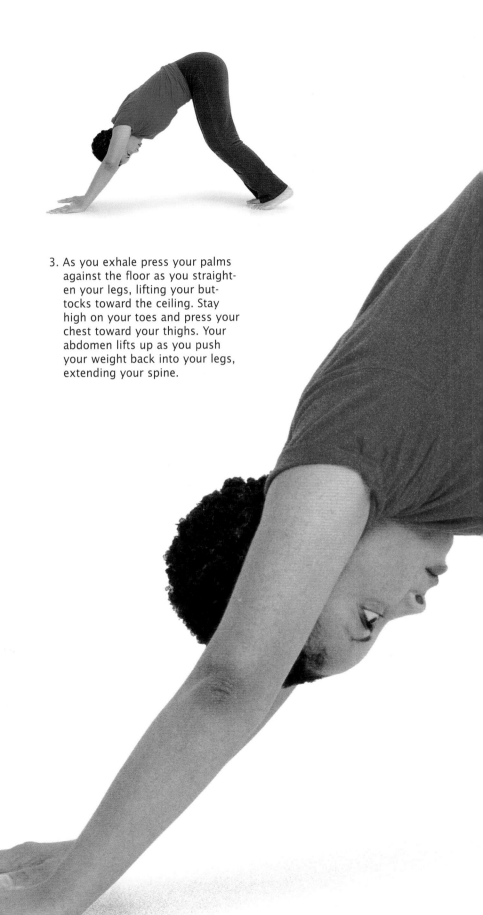

1. Begin in The Cat pose, on all fours. Spread your fingers wide apart and keep your hands pressed against the floor beneath your shoulders. Your arms are straight. Your back is parallel to the floor. Tuck your toes under.

2. Inhale.

3. As you exhale press your palms against the floor as you straighten your legs, lifting your buttocks toward the ceiling. Stay high on your toes and press your chest toward your thighs. Your abdomen lifts up as you push your weight back into your legs, extending your spine.

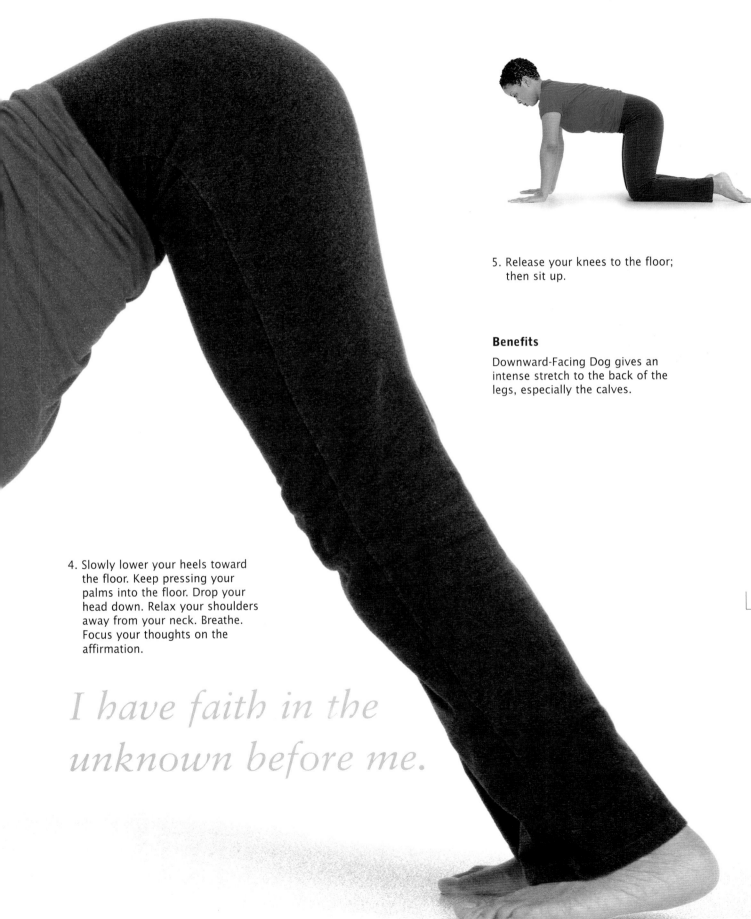

5. Release your knees to the floor;
   then sit up.

Benefits

Downward-Facing Dog gives an intense stretch to the back of the legs, especially the calves.

4. Slowly lower your heels toward the floor. Keep pressing your palms into the floor. Drop your head down. Relax your shoulders away from your neck. Breathe. Focus your thoughts on the affirmation.

I have faith in the unknown before me.

19) HEAD TO KNEE POSE

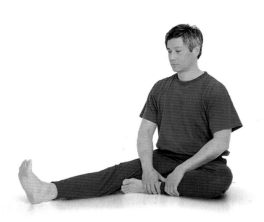
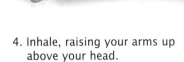

1. Sit up straight on the floor with your legs extended out in front of you.

2. Bend your left knee and place the sole of your left foot against your right inner thigh.

3. Flex your right foot.

4. Inhale, raising your arms up above your head.

5. Exhale, bending at your hips, lowering your chest and head toward your right knee.

6. Bring your hands down to your right calf, ankle, or foot, wherever you can comfortably reach.

7. Hold the pose while breathing. Focus your thoughts on the affirmation.

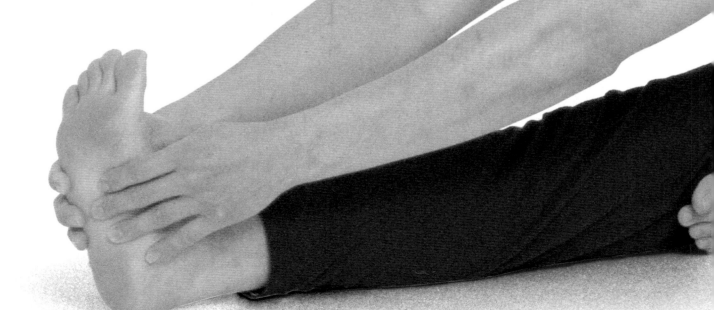

Everything I need I possess in this moment.

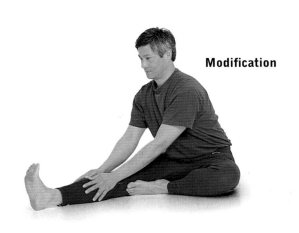

Modification

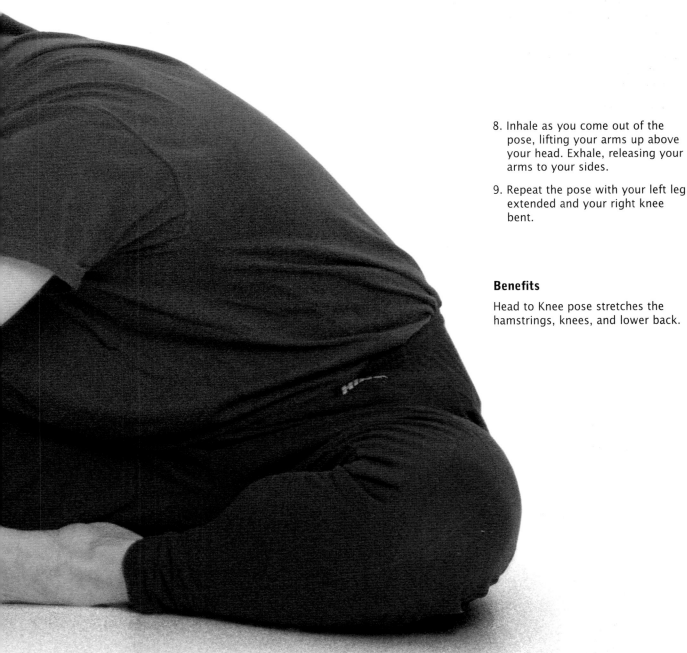

8. Inhale as you come out of the pose, lifting your arms up above your head. Exhale, releasing your arms to your sides.

9. Repeat the pose with your left leg extended and your right knee bent.

Benefits

Head to Knee pose stretches the hamstrings, knees, and lower back.

20) SEATED FORWARD BEND

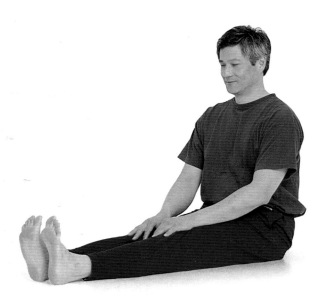

1. Sit on the floor with your legs extended out in front of you.

2. Rotate your ankles, flexing and stretching them to loosen them up.

3. Sit up straight and flex your feet.

4. Inhale, raising your arms up above your head.

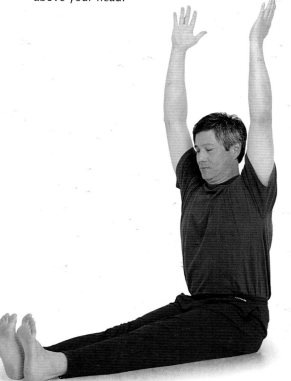

5. Exhale, bending at the hips, lowering your chest toward your knees. Keep your spine straight as you do this.

6. Place your hands on your calves, ankles, or feet, wherever you can comfortably reach.

7. Keep your feet flexed. Hold the pose while breathing. Focus your thoughts on the affirmation.

I move forward with patience.

8. Inhale, raising your arms straight up above your head as you sit up.

9. Exhale, lowering your arms to your sides.

Benefits

Seated Forward Bend helps limber the hamstrings and lower back.

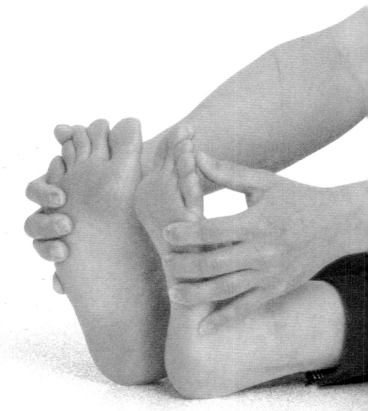

GENTLE YOGA FOR HEALING

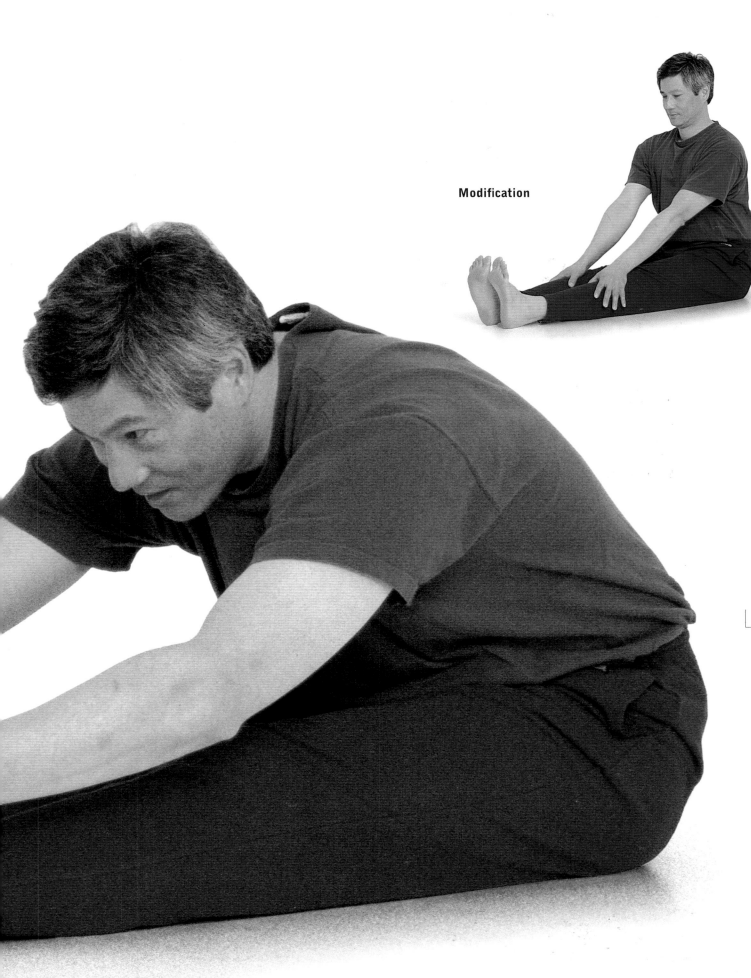

Modification

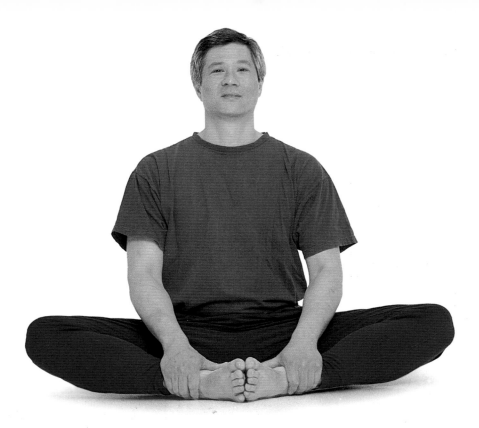

1. Sit up straight. Place the bottoms of your feet together, pulling them in toward your groin. Your knees should be out to your sides.

2. Inhale.

My spirit is as gentle as a butterfly.

Modification

- Lean your back against a wall for more support. If your knees are not able to lower down to the floor, place folded blankets or pillows under the thighs for support and apply a gentle downward pressure on the thighs.

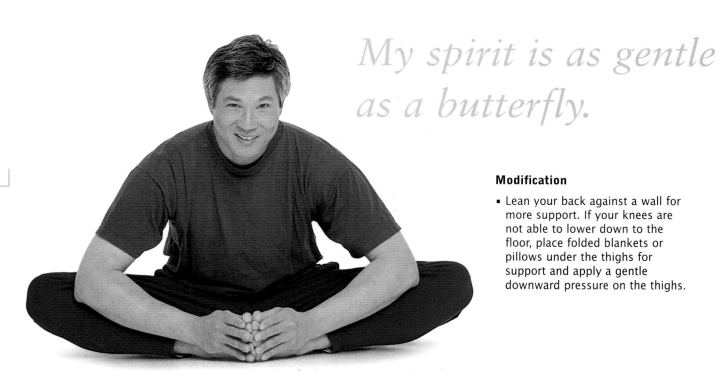

3. As you exhale, lean forward. Clasp your feet and begin pressing your forearms into your calves and knees, gently pushing your knees toward the floor.

4. Hold the pose while continuing to press your knees down. Breathe. Focus your thoughts on the affirmation.

5. Inhale, sitting back up and releasing your knees.

Benefits

The Butterfly pose works to gently open the pelvis.

22) INNER-THIGH STRETCH

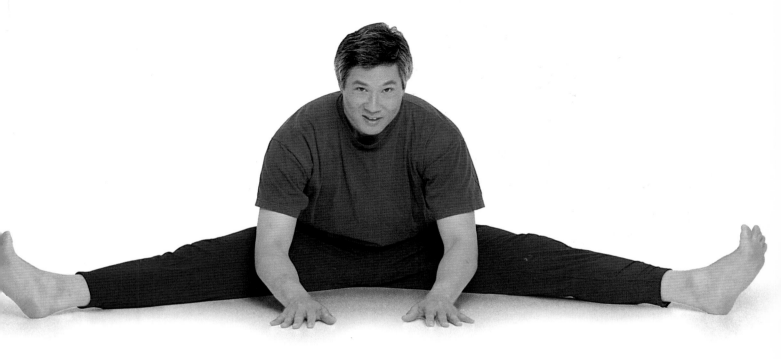

1. Sit on the floor with your legs extended out in front of you.

2. Spread your legs out into a V position, as wide as is comfortable.

3. Flex your feet (bend your knees slightly if you like).

4. Inhale, sitting up straight.

5. Exhale and lean forward as you slowly walk your hands out away from you. You should be lowering your chest toward the floor.

6. Breathe. Focus your thoughts on the affirmation.

Nonresistance gives me peace.

7. When you feel ready, walk your hands back up and slide your legs together in front of you.

Benefits

Inner-Thigh Stretch improves inner-thigh flexibility and loosens the hip joints.

23) ROCK THE BABY

1. Sit up straight on the floor with your legs extended forward.

2. Raise your left leg and bend it toward you.

3. Place both arms around your leg as if you were cradling a baby—your left foot is in the bend of your right elbow and your knee is in the bend of your left elbow.

4. If you can reach easily, interlace your fingers.

5. Gently rock your leg from side to side. Focus your thoughts on the affirmation.

I gently open to my inner wisdom.

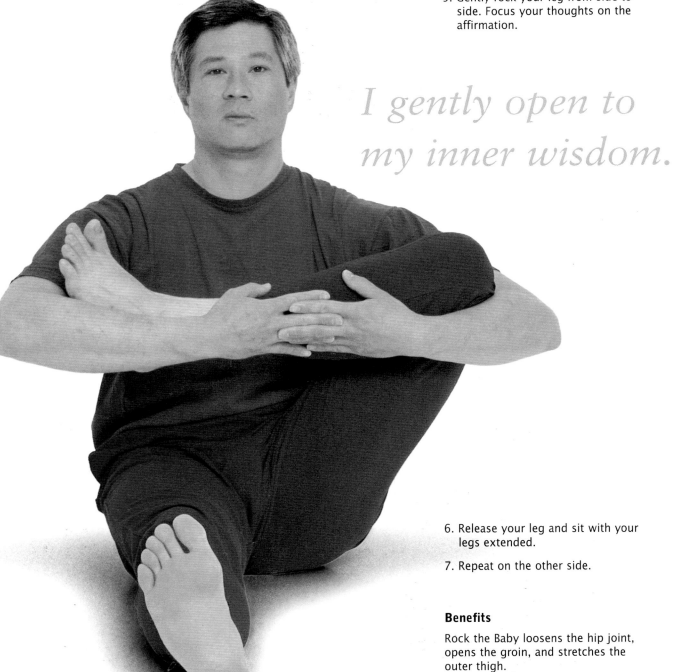

6. Release your leg and sit with your legs extended.

7. Repeat on the other side.

Benefits

Rock the Baby loosens the hip joint, opens the groin, and stretches the outer thigh.

24) GENTLE SPINAL TWIST

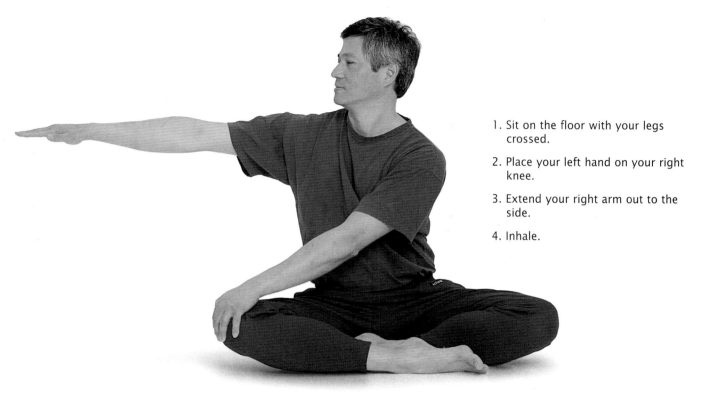

1. Sit on the floor with your legs crossed.

2. Place your left hand on your right knee.

3. Extend your right arm out to the side.

4. Inhale.

5. As you exhale, twist to the right bringing your right arm around behind your back and resting your right hand on your left inner thigh, if you can reach that far.

6. Look over your right shoulder. Breathe. Focus your thoughts on the affirmation.

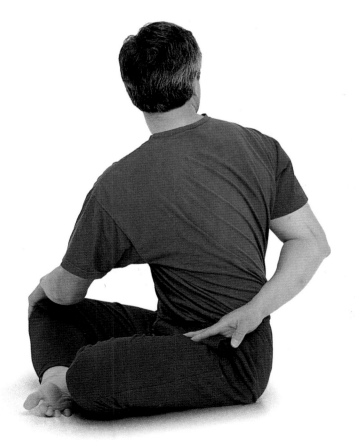

I let go of the past with forgiveness.

7. Exhale, releasing the pose.

8. Repeat the pose, twisting to the left.

Benefits

Gentle Spinal Twist increases elasticity of the spine.

25) SITTING BOAT

1. Lie on your back with your legs together and your arms beside your body.

2. Take a deep breath.

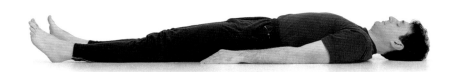

3. As you exhale, raise both legs and your upper body until you are balancing on your hips.

4. Extend your arms forward, parallel to the floor, reaching toward your toes.

5. Hold the pose—at first, for just a moment; then gradually work up to holding it for several breaths. Focus your thoughts on the affirmation.

My faith in life gives me inner strength.

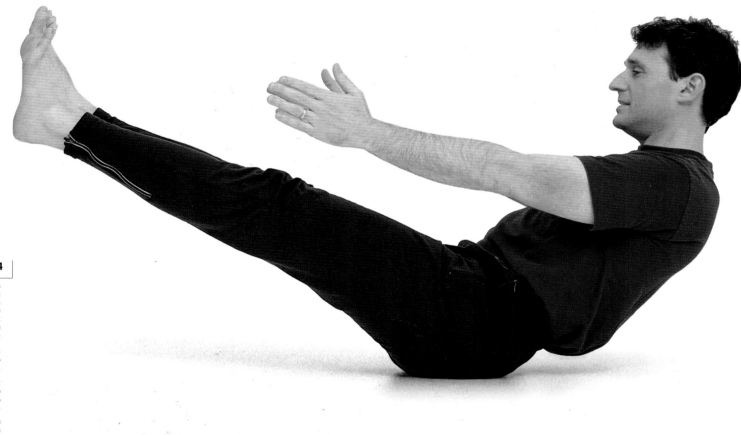

6. Release, lie down, and relax.

Modification

If you have strain in your lower back, then keep your knees bent in the pose.

Benefits

Sitting Boat pose helps to strengthen the stomach muscles.

26) LITTLE BOAT (HUGGING KNEES)

1. Lie on your back. Bring your knees in toward your chest.

2. Wrap your arms around your knees and legs, hugging them in toward your chest. Keep your chin slightly tucked so your neck is lengthened on the floor.

3. Hold the position and breathe. Focus your thoughts on the affirmation.

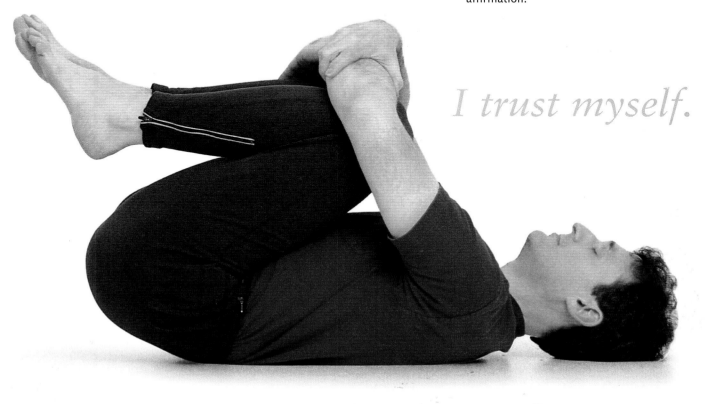

I trust myself.

4. Release your legs and arms so that you are lying on the floor.

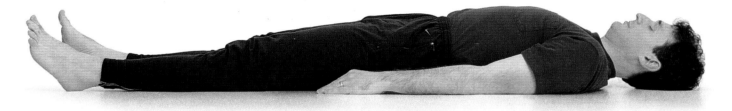

Benefits

Little Boat pose releases the lower back and lengthens the spine.

27) GENTLE PELVIC ROCKING

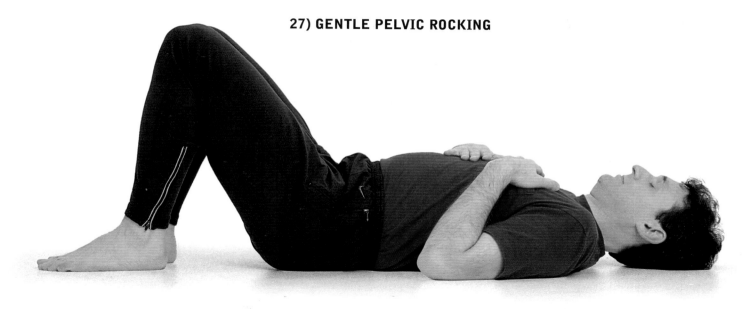

1. Lie on your back.

2. Bend your knees, placing your feet flat on the floor. Draw them in toward your buttocks so that your knees are pointed upward, side by side.

3. Inhale, pressing your lower back into the floor. Tighten your buttocks and lift one or two of your lowest vertebra off the floor, just lifting your tailbone slightly. Focus your thoughts on the affirmation.

I like myself unconditionally.

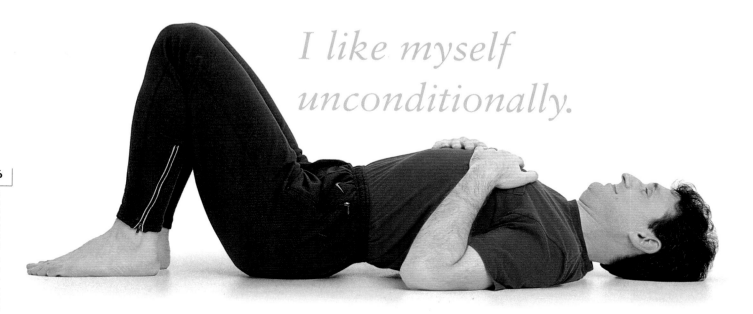

4. Exhale, pressing your tailbone back down toward the floor so that your lower back arches. Focus your thoughts on the affirmation.

5. Inhale, pressing your lower back in the floor, tightening your buttocks, and lifting your tailbone slightly again. Focus your thoughts on the affirmation.

6. Exhale, releasing your tailbone allowing your lower back to arch. Repeat the affirmation.

7. Continue rocking your pelvis gently and slowly 9–10 times.

Benefits

Gentle Pelvic Rocking increases the strength and suppleness of the pelvic region while toning the buttocks muscle.

GENTLE YOGA FOR HEALING

28) SLANT BOARD (DESK)

1. Lie on your back and place your feet flat on the floor, drawing them in toward your buttocks so that your knees are pointed upward.

2. Inhale, and press your lower back into the floor.

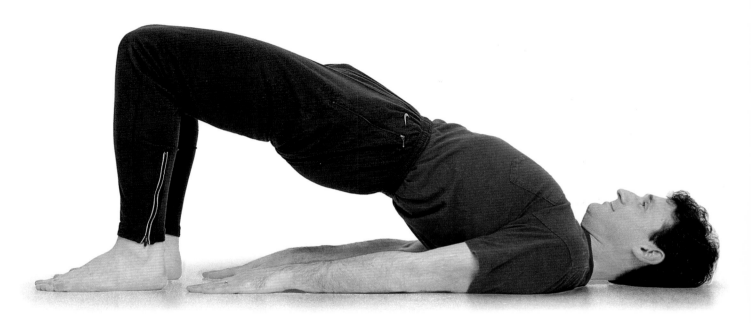

3. Exhale, lifting your tailbone and lifting your vertebrae slowly, your thighs lifting up so that you create a slanted surface, a straight line from your knees to your shoulders. Your chin should be tucked into your chest.

4. Hold the pose while breathing. Focus your thoughts on the affirmation.

Honesty is my commitment to myself.

5. Exhale, coming back down slowly, one vertebra at a time, beginning with your upper back and ending with your lower back, pressing into the floor.

Benefits

Slant Board pose stretches the spine and releases neck tension. It reverses the pull of gravity, allowing blood to flow toward the chest, neck, and head.

29) THE ARCH

1. Lie on your back with your knees bent and your feet flat on the floor. Place your feet hip-width apart, drawn in toward your buttocks with your knees pointed upward.

2. Inhale, pressing your lower back into the floor.

3. Exhale, lifting your tailbone and continuing to lift up into an arch. Press your feet into the floor, lifting your thighs and stomach up high. Clasp your hands underneath your back, and interlace your fingers. Straighten your arms. Your chin should be tucked.

4. Hold the pose while breathing. Focus your thoughts on the affirmation.

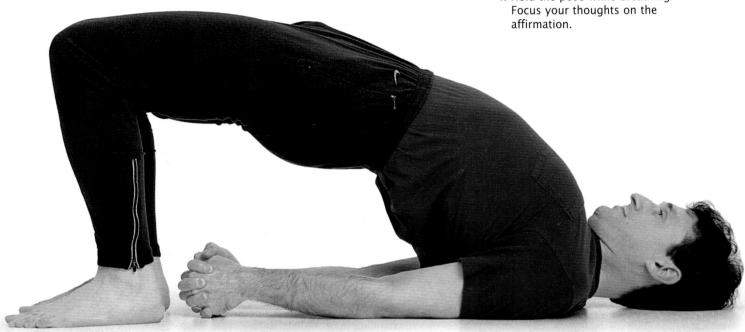

I am uplifted as I live in truth.

GENTLE YOGA FOR HEALING

5. Exhale, releasing your hands and coming down one vertebra at a time from the top of your shoulders all the way down to your tailbone.

6. Take a deep breath and release it.

7. Pull your knees into your chest for a moment. Then extend your legs and relax.

Benefits

The Arch increases flexibility in the spine and shoulders and develops strength in the lower back and stomach. It also releases tension in the abdomen.

30) KNEE HUG SPINAL TWIST

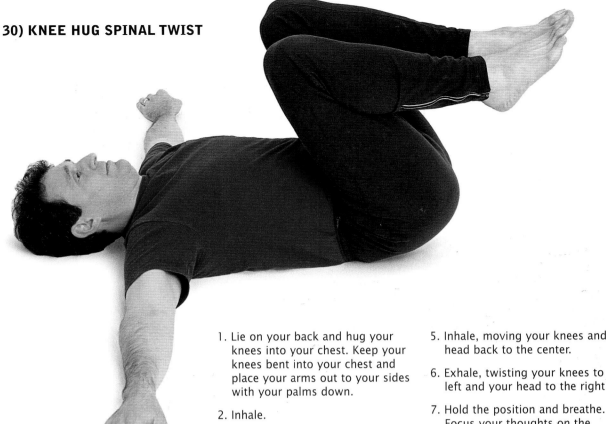

1. Lie on your back and hug your knees into your chest. Keep your knees bent into your chest and place your arms out to your sides with your palms down.

2. Inhale.

3. Exhale, twisting your knees to the right as you turn your head to the left.

4. Hold the position and breathe. Focus your thoughts on the affirmation.

5. Inhale, moving your knees and head back to the center.

6. Exhale, twisting your knees to the left and your head to the right.

7. Hold the position and breathe. Focus your thoughts on the affirmation.

8. Inhale, moving your knees and head back to the center.

9. Release your legs and lie flat. Relax.

Everywhere I turn I see beauty.

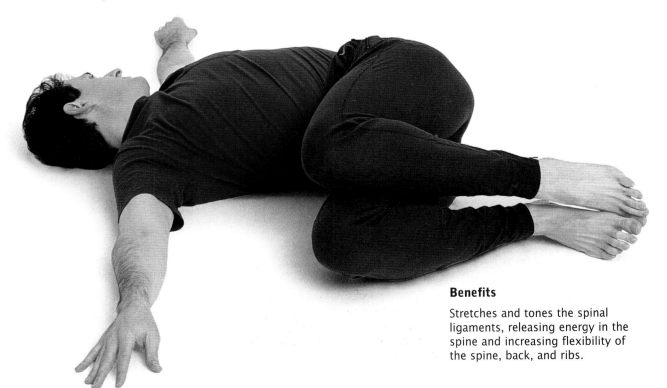

Benefits

Stretches and tones the spinal ligaments, releasing energy in the spine and increasing flexibility of the spine, back, and ribs.

31) HALF PLOUGH

Caution: Do not attempt the half plough if you have high blood pressure, have a sinus infection, have a loose retina, are menstruating, or have a weak or injured neck or lower back.

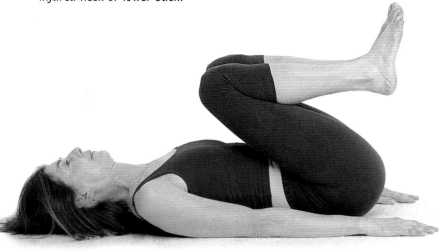

1. Lie on your back, placing your arms along the sides of your body with your palms facing down and your legs together.

2. Bring your knees up to your abdomen. Then, straighten them toward the ceiling.

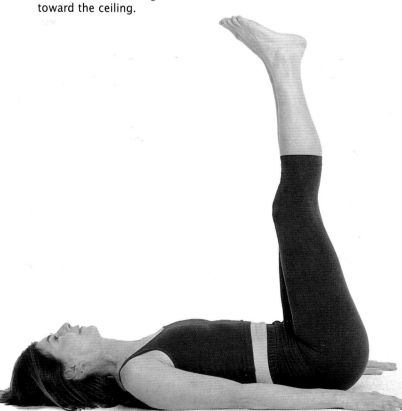

3. Exhale, pushing against the floor with your hands as you lift your torso.

4. Raise your hips off the floor and extend your feet behind your head until your legs are parallel to the floor. Support your lower back with your hands. Your chin should be tucked into your chest.

5. Breathe evenly as you hold the pose. Focus your thoughts on the affirmation.

I am grateful for this moment of life.

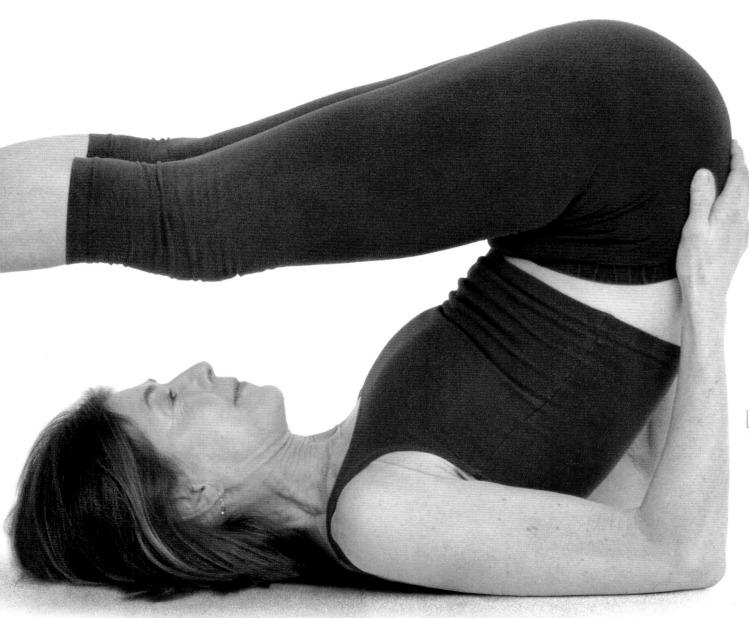

6. Exhale and slowly lower your hips. Return your legs to perpendicular position.

7. Continue exhaling as you slowly lower your legs to the floor.

Benefits

Half Plough pose promotes spinal flexibility and deep relaxation of all the muscles. It improves the functioning of the internal organs by supplying them with extra blood.

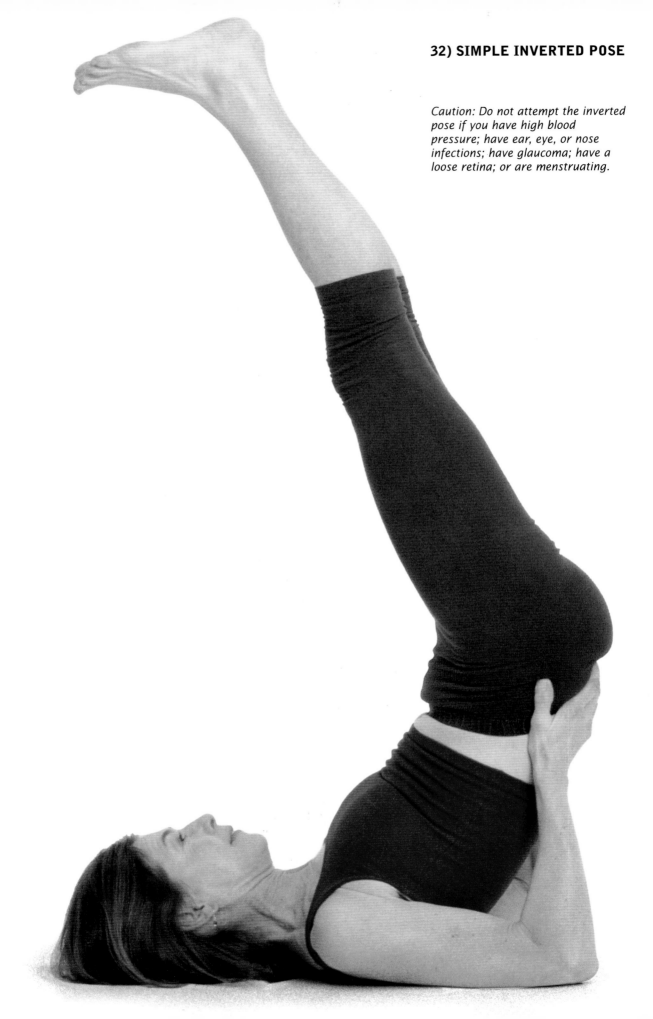

32) SIMPLE INVERTED POSE

Caution: Do not attempt the inverted pose if you have high blood pressure; have ear, eye, or nose infections; have glaucoma; have a loose retina; or are menstruating.

1. Lie on your back.

2. Inhale and slowly raise your legs up so that they are perpendicular to the floor.

3. Keeping your legs in a vertical position, slowly raise your hips until you can support them with your hands. Keep your thumbs just under your hip joints and place your elbows on the floor about a foot apart; if your elbows are too far apart, they will not give adequate support to your body, which is resting on them. Your neck is free. The weight of the pose should be on your elbows, not your neck. Keep your legs straight and toes pointed.

4. Hold the pose while breathing. Focus your thoughts on the affirmation.

I accept all of my feelings as a part of myself.

5. Exhale, slowly lowering your hips and returning your legs to a perpendicular position.

6. Continue exhaling and slowly lower your legs to the floor.

Modification

If you are unable to do Simple Inverted Pose, substitute Leg Inversion against the Wall.

Benefits

Simple Inverted Pose helps reverse the pull of gravity. It relaxes the legs by relieving pressure. It allows blood to flow into the upper body, giving the glands and organs a lift.

33) LEG INVERSION AGAINST THE WALL

If you are unable to do the Simple Inverted Pose, this is a great substitute.

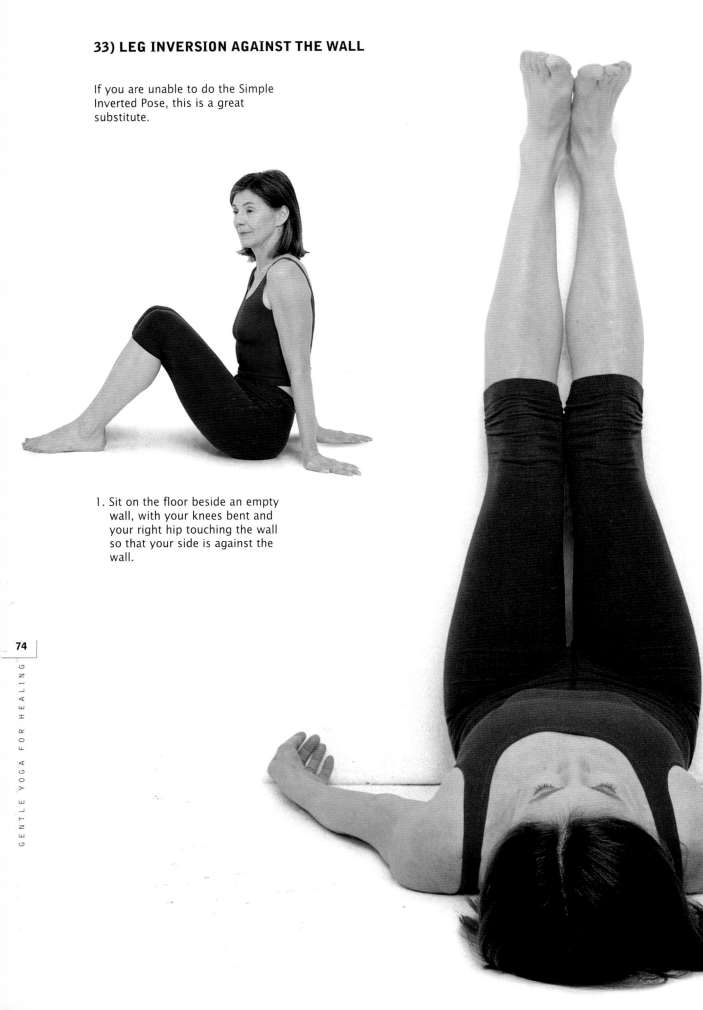

1. Sit on the floor beside an empty wall, with your knees bent and your right hip touching the wall so that your side is against the wall.

2. Slide your legs up the wall as you turn your body toward the wall.

3. Keep your buttocks against the wall and lie with your torso on the floor and your legs elevated against the wall.

4. Straighten your legs.

5. Hold the pose and breathe. Focus your thoughts on the affirmation.

As I relax, I gain insight, clarity, and ease.

6. Bend your knees and lower your legs beside the wall. Move away from the wall and lie down on your back.

Benefits

Leg Inversion against the Wall pose relaxes the legs and feet by relieving pressure.

Modification

Place a pillow under your head and buttocks for more support.

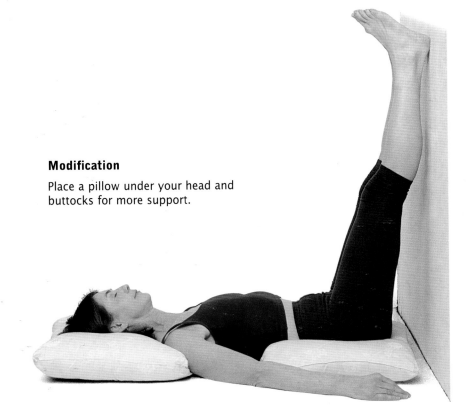
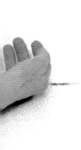

34) FISH

This pose is a counterpose to the Simple Inverted Pose and Half Plough, bending your neck and head in the opposite direction. You need strong back muscles to hold the lift of your upper back in the arched Fish pose.

1. Lie on your back.

2. Place your hands under your buttocks, palms up, and inhale.

3. Exhale as you press your elbows and forearms into the floor and lift your sternum or breastbone away from the floor.

4. Arch your back. Stretch your neck backward, resting the crown of your head on the floor.

5. Hold the pose while breathing evenly. Focus your thoughts on the affirmation.

I breathe easily as I release control.

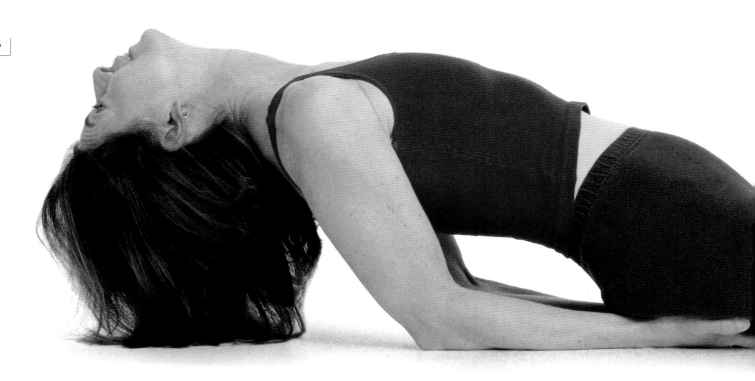

6. Slowly lower your shoulders and neck to the ground. Relax.

Benefits

Fish pose relieves a stiff neck, opens the breathing cavity, opens the shoulders, and relieves tension in the throat.

Modification

If you are a beginner, have back pain, or have a weak upper back, substitute The Camel (Preparation) pose.

Caution: If your neck hurts, lower your shoulders and neck to the ground and release the pose. Do not push yourself beyond your limits.

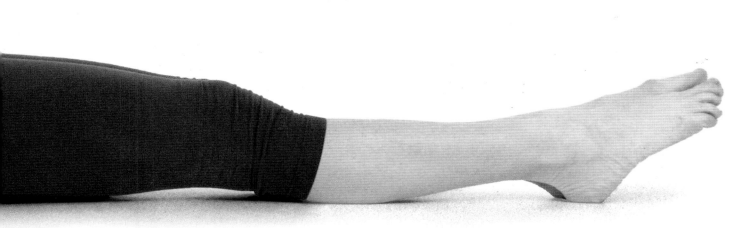

35) CORPSE POSE

1. Lie on your back and gently close your eyes.

2. Place your feet and legs slightly apart.

3. Place your arms along the sides of your body with your palms facing up. Make sure your teeth are slightly parted so that your jaw is relaxed.

4. Start taking some deep breaths. In the pose your body should resemble a corpse, lying still and relaxed. Focus your thoughts on the affirmation.

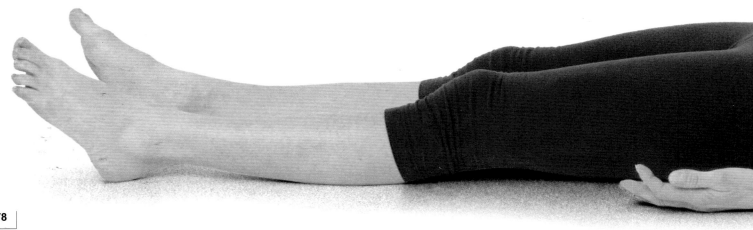

I allow myself to relax completely.

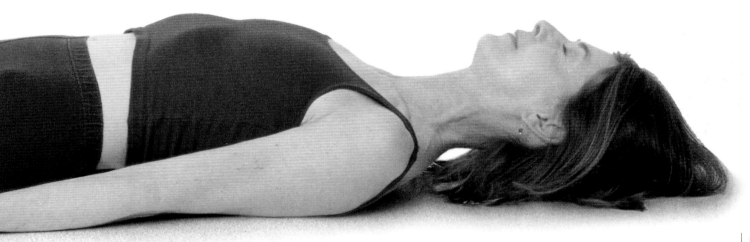

6. Stay in this position for 5–10 minutes.

Benefits

Corpse Pose is the basic pose of relaxation that is done at the end of each hatha yoga session. It helps relieve the body of tension, and it relieves the body and mind of fatigue. It relaxes, rejuvenates, and replenishes the mind and body.

Four-Week Routine

WEEK ONE

Day 1   Straight standing posture
Warm up
Side stretch
Angle stretch
Corpse

Day 2   Straight standing posture
Warm up
Side stretch
Angle stretch
Triangle
Corpse

Day 3   Straight standing posture
Warm up
Side stretch
Angle stretch
Triangle
Squat
Corpse

Day 4   Warm up
Side stretch
Angle stretch
Triangle
Squat
Warrior
Corpse

Day 5   Warm up
Side stretch
Angle stretch
Warrior
Chair
Tree
Corpse

Day 6   Warm up
Side stretch
Triangle
Warrior
Chair
Tree
Corpse

Day 7   Rest

WEEK TWO

Day 8   Warm up
Tree
Sitting mountain
Child's pose
Cobra
Cat
Corpse

Day 9   Warm up
Side stretch
Angle pose
Sitting mountain
Cobra
Backward bend
Child's pose
Corpse

Day 10   Warm up
Mountain
Cobra
Lying down boat
Cat
Backward bend
Child's pose
Downward dog
Corpse

Day 11   Warm up
Sitting mountain
Child's pose
Cobra
Lying boat
Cat
Head to knee
Forward bend
Corpse

Day 12   Warm up
Child's pose
Cat
Backward bend
Camel preparation
Downward dog
Head to knee
Forward bend
Corpse

Day 13   Warm up
Child's pose
Cobra
Lying boat
Cat
Backward bend
Camel
Downward dog
Head to knee
Forward bend
Corpse

Day 14   Rest

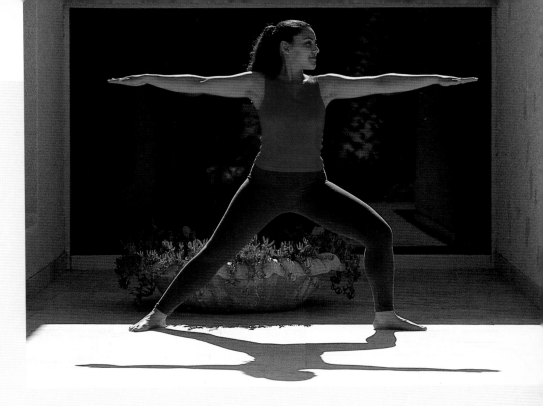

WEEK THREE

Day 15 Warm up
Head to knee
Sitting forward bend
Butterfly
Inner thigh stretch
Rock the baby
Gentle spinal twist
Corpse

Day 16 Warm up
Sitting forward bend
Butterfly
Inner thigh stretch
Rock the baby
Sitting boat
Little boat
Knee hugging spinal twist
Corpse

Day 17 Warm up
Head to knee
Forward bend
Butterfly
Inner thigh
Rock the baby
Gentle spinal twist
Sitting boat
Gentle pelvic rocking
Corpse

Day 18 Warm up
Side stretch
Chair
Tree
Forward bend
Butterfly
Inner thigh
Gentle pelvic rocking
Slant board
Knee hug spinal twist
Corpse

Day 19 Warm up
Downward dog
Child's pose
Head to knee
Forward bend
Gentle pelvic rocking
Slant board
Arch
Knee hug spinal twist
Leg inversion against wall
Corpse

Day 20 Warm up
Inner thigh stretch
Rock the baby
Gentle spinal twist
Sitting boat
Gentle pelvic rocking
Slant board
Arch
Half plough
Leg inversions against wall
Corpse

Day 21 Rest

WEEK FOUR

Day 22 Warm up
Side stretch
Angle stretch
Triangle
Squat
Warrior
Sitting mountain
Child's pose
Corpse

Day 23 Warm up
Downward dog
Mountain
Backward bend
Camel
Child's pose
Cobra
Lying-down boat
Cat
Corpse

Day 24 Mountain
Child's pose
Cobra
Lying-down boat
Sitting boat
Little boat
Gentle pelvic rocking
Slant
Arch
Knee hugging spinal twist
Corpse

Day 25 Warm up
Side stretch
Angle stretch
Triangle
Chair
Tree
Sitting forward bend
Half plough
Simple inverted pose
Fish
Corpse

Day 26 Warm up
Side stretch
Triangle
Tree
Cat
Backward bend
Camel
Downward dog
Child's pose
Leg inversion against wall
Corpse

Day 27 Warm up
Cat
Downward dog
Forward bend
Butterfly
Inner thigh
Sitting boat
Lying boat
Cobra
Child's pose
Knee hugging spinal twist
Half plough
Simple inverted pose
Fish
Corpse

Day 28 Rest

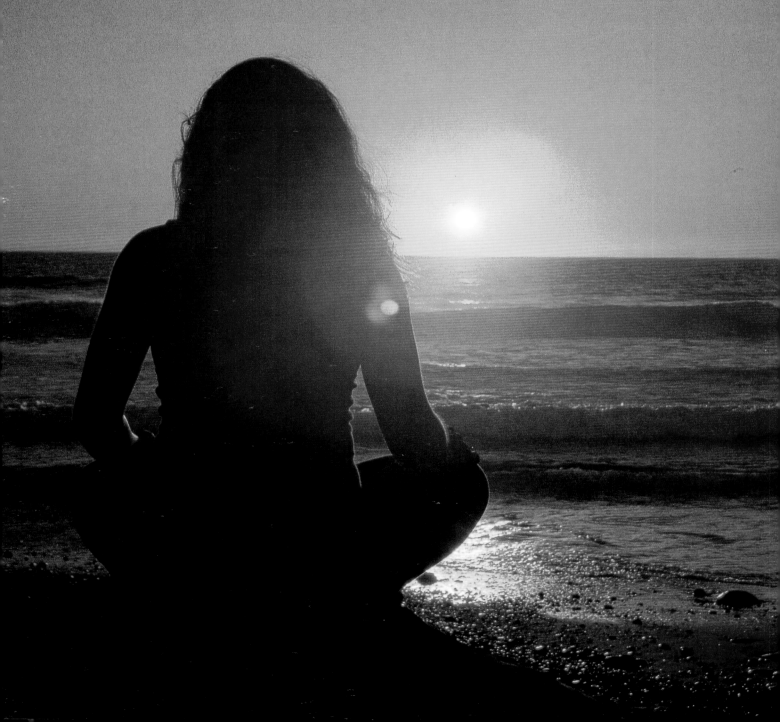

Relaxation,

CHAPTER FIVE

Meditation, and Prayer

Everybody wants to feel good. We all want to feel safe and loved and accepted. We want to feel at peace. Yet so often we find ourselves feeling the opposite. Busy hectic schedules, projects to complete, conflicts with co-workers or family members, health challenges, unpaid bills, unmet goals, disappointments, driving through traffic—there are numerous situations that keep people feeling uptight and tense.

Yoga teaches that peace begins within. When we quiet our mind and body, we can more readily access our intuition and connect to our divine nature. We find meaning beyond the physical realm, which helps put things in perspective. We learn to balance all the daily exterior stimulation with our own interior stillness. It is inside our own heart and soul that we find the resources for solving our problems and moving toward our highest good.

Learning to have faith has not been an easy process for me. I am amazed at how often fear can creep into my mind. I often find myself resisting

and holding onto my defenses, rather than yielding to the circumstances of my life with trust and faith. And so I use my yoga practices to help bring myself back inside to that place of stillness where peace can be found.

The techniques offered in this chapter—relaxation, meditation, and prayer—are the tools I use to get in touch with my inner guidance. As I learn to relax and simply stay receptive, I become conscious of an intuitive knowing that is somehow linked to a spiritual presence that guides my life. I do not always feel this presence. But when I make time for relaxation, meditation, and prayer I do begin to feel at peace and I actually feel a calming and healing energy rise up within me from the depths of my being. It is like opening a door to the grace of God, flowing through my life. That door is always there waiting to be opened, but I am so easily distracted; life can get very busy. Yet when I allow myself to simply rest in stillness, even for a few moments, I am rewarded with clarity and ease. I am reminded of my desire to grow spiritually and my willingness to be open and receptive to life's lessons. This inward, quiet time helps remove my resistance to opening my heart and listening within. It helps awaken my faith with an peaceful inner consciousness that sees beyond the outer appearances of the world.

Relaxation

One of the nicest parts of yoga class is the relaxation period after practicing the postures. My students love this time, and so do I. It is a time to lie down in the Corpse Pose, allow your body to completely let go of all tension, and simply be. No doing, no performing. Just being.

Occasionally I have beginning students who have a difficult time letting go into relaxation. They do not know how to release the holding and tension in their bodies. Through yoga, they start becoming aware of tensions they never realized they had. Change begins with awareness. Before you know that something is out of balance it is hard to make a change.

These students remind me of the first time I discovered how much stored tension I carried in my own body. I first became aware of my need for relaxation when I was seventeen and decided to take some massage classes offered at a local health club. The instructor asked me if I had ever had a professional massage; when I said no, he told me that getting one was a prerequisite for the class. He said, "You must know how to receive before you can give." Being massaged was my first experience with getting in touch with my body. That first massage gave me an awareness of how much tension I was holding. The therapist working on me kept telling me to let go and relax—but I had no idea of how to do that. That first massage was an eye-opener.

I was still living with my parents at the time and my home environment was stressful. My father had been an alcoholic, and he was dying of cancer. I was accustomed to living with a high level of stress, and carrying accumulated tension in my body and mind—so much so, that I did not even notice it. After another year, during which I left home for college, my father died, and I was faced with making choices for my future, I decided to go to massage school to learn more about helping my body relax. A few years later, I began my studies in hatha yoga, which further enhanced my ability to release tension from my body and mind.

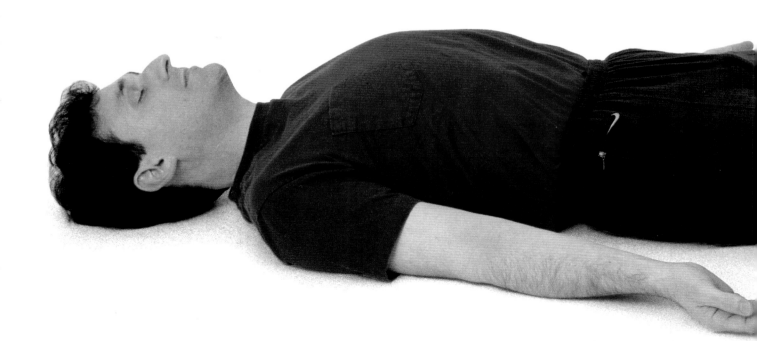

Relaxation is a skill that anyone can learn—I learned it, and so can you. Learning to relax is not difficult, but it does require a conscious effort, patience, and, like learning any skill, such as playing the piano, the more you practice the better skilled you become.

Some people say, "Oh, I relax by watching TV," or "I relax on the golf course," but this is not the kind of relaxation I am talking about. The kind of relaxation we need in order to heal our bodies is a total relaxation of body, mind, and spirit. Total relaxation requires being rather than doing. It is a period of rest and tranquility that creates a calming effect on the mind and releases tension from the body. Practicing complete relaxation for even 10 minutes a day relieves fatigue, reduces stress, and revitalizes the body. It is a period of rejuvenation and replenishment.

This is different from sleep. During sleep, you do not necessarily let go of the tensions in your body. In fact, studies have shown that the muscles do not relax at all as you sleep—the amount of muscular tension you fall asleep with is the amount of muscular tension you wake up with. Even if you wake up feeling refreshed after a night's sleep, it does not mean that the accumu-

lated tension of weeks and years has been washed away.

Relaxation is an acquired skill. Complete relaxation requires focusing on the body and mind to relieve tension and create a feeling of peace and ease. When practiced regularly, relaxation allows us to prevent the body from building up and accumulating tension. It gives us an awareness of where we are holding tension in our body and how to release that tension.

We can actually learn to shed our stress—bodies lengthen, faces soften, hearts open. Deep relaxation allows for greater receptivity to healing. Developing this skill is one of the safest and most effective ways to manage stress, relieve anxiety, ease pain, and regain peace of mind.

PRACTICING RELAXATION

Relaxation can be practiced whenever you have ten or fifteen minutes to lie down in a quiet place, but the ideal time is right after you have practiced your hatha yoga postures because you have already begun to release tension in your joints and muscles through stretching your body. Relaxation helps to release tensions not only in your body but

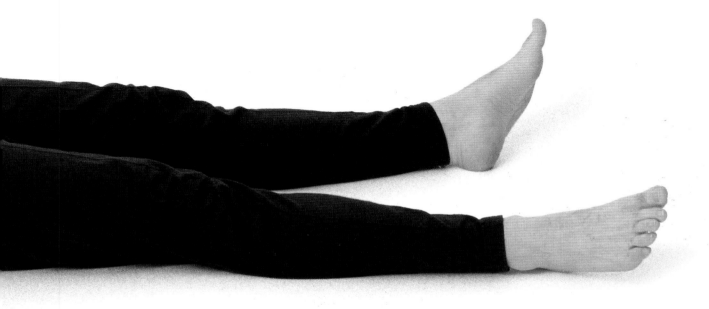

also your mind—it is a time to let go completely and relax both physically and mentally.

When practicing the relaxation techniques in this chapter, read the instructions over once before trying them. Then ask a friend to read this to you while you are lying down or, better yet, tape your own voice and listen to it after you do your yoga poses. If you like, you can play some soft soothing music in the background. As you become proficient at using these techniques, it will require less and less time for you to reach relaxation. Your body will respond positively each time you practice.

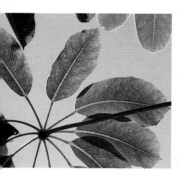

Basic Relaxation Position

The basic position for practicing relaxation is lying down on your back. A warm soft blanket will improve your comfort and ability to relax in this position. Lie down with your knees bent and your feet flat on the floor, and gently press your lower back into the floor. It is important for your knees to be bent because it helps to properly align your lower back. Put a pillow under your knees and thighs so you are not using your muscles to keep your knees bent. If you want to lie flat, begin with your knees bent and extend your legs one at a time without arching your back off the floor. Allow your legs to separate slightly. Place your arms down at your sides, slightly away from your body with your palms face up. Pull your shoulders down toward your feet. Gently extend the curve of your neck so that your chin comes down slightly. Make sure your teeth are slightly parted so that your jaw is relaxed. Close your eyes.

Tensing-Relaxing Technique

1. Begin taking some long deep breaths. After four or five breaths, bring your awareness down to your feet, curling your toes and flexing your feet. Hold this for three seconds and as you exhale, let go and relax your feet.

2. Now bring your awareness to your legs. As you inhale, squeeze and tighten your legs. Hold this for three seconds; as you exhale, release and relax your legs. Take a deep breath and release.

3. Bring your awareness to your buttocks. As you inhale, squeeze and tighten your buttocks. Hold this for three seconds; as you exhale, release and relax your buttocks. Take another deep breath and release further.

4. Bring your awareness to your abdominal area. As you inhale, tighten your abdomen and the internal organs. Hold this for three seconds; as you exhale, release the abdominal area and allow the stomach to be soft and relaxed. Take another deep breath and release more deeply.

5. Now bring your awareness to your chest area. As you inhale, press your shoulder blades into the floor while lifting and tensing your chest. Hold this for three seconds; as you exhale, release your shoulder blades and relax your chest.

6. Bring your awareness to your shoulders. As you inhale, gently press your shoulder blades down to the floor, opening the chest. Then think of gently pulling your shoulder down, away from your ears and toward your feet. Take a deep breath and release.

7. Next, bring your awareness to your arms and hands. As you inhale, tighten your arms and squeeze your hands into fists. Hold this for three seconds. Exhale, release the arms, relax the hands, and allow them to lie with palms up like gloves lying on a table, empty and still.

8. Now bring your awareness to your face. As you inhale, tighten your face, crinkle your forehead, clench your teeth—make a prune face. Hold this for three seconds. As you exhale, relax your face, release your jaw, and enjoy the tingling sensation of all the tension leaving your face. Continue taking deep long breaths, focusing on your exhalations and allowing your body to relax more and more.

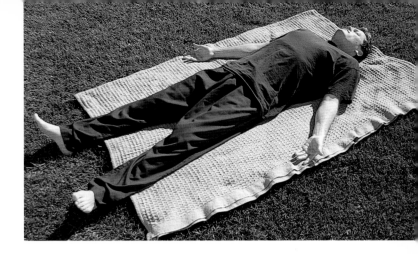

Relaxation Breathing Technique

1. Play some calm, soothing music in the background. Lie down for relaxation. Close your eyes. Mentally scan your body for tension. Notice if your neck, shoulders, or back feel tense. Take your time. If you notice any tightness, do not judge it to be negative. Just notice where you are feeling tension. You are checking in with your body in a loving way.

2. After you have scanned your entire body for tension, bring your awareness to your breath. Imagine that you are able to breathe into each part of your body, helping it to relax and open. Visualize the air you are breathing in traveling to each body part. Begin with your feet. As you inhale, visualize the air traveling all the way down to your feet, helping them relax. As you exhale, all tension leaves your feet. Inhale and visualize the air traveling to your legs. Your legs become warm and relaxed as you inhale. As you exhale, all tension leaves the legs. Work your way up the body. Each time you inhale, you breathe in relaxation. Each time you exhale, you release tension. Take as long as you want at each body part, breathing into the area and helping it to relax.

3. If you come to an area that feels particularly tight, keep breathing into that area. Visualize the breath going straight to that area helping it to relax and open. With every exhalation, tension leaves your body.

As you work your way up, your entire body opens and widens. Your breathing is slow and even. You are relaxed.

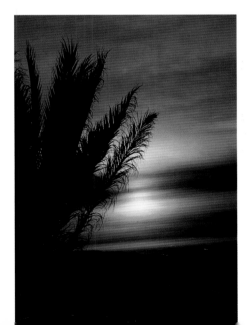

Relaxation Visualization Technique

I often use visualizations during the relaxation period to assist with the process of letting go and healing. The following is a visualization script on healing affirmation and relaxation.

1. Lie down on your back. Start with your knees bent and your feet flat on the floor, gently pressing your lower back into the floor. Place a pillow under your knees for support or, if you want to lie flat, extend your legs one at a time without arching the back off the floor. Allow the legs to separate slightly.

2. Place your arms down at your sides, with palms faced up in an attitude of receiving the life energy that circulates in the air around us.

3. Make sure your teeth are slightly parted so that your jaw is relaxed. Relax your shoulders down toward your feet.

4. Close your eyes. Start taking some deep, long breaths—breathing in peace and relaxation, exhaling and releasing all tension, all anxieties. Continue taking deep, long breaths. Your arms and legs are warm and heavy. Allow yourself to relax.

5. Now visualize a warm, healing light shining above your body. This warm healing light is shining down on your body, sending love and warmth, sending healing energy to every atom and every cell in your body. And all you have to do is allow yourself to receive it. Breathe in the light. This warm, healing light is calming and healing your entire body. All fatigue is leaving. Your body energy flows freely and evenly. And now silently say to yourself, "I allow myself to relax completely. I allow myself to relax completely." Feel your body opening and releasing all tension as it relaxes. The floor beneath you is supporting you completely—breathing in, breathing

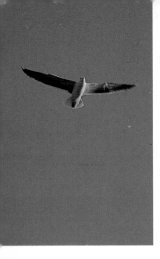

out. Allow yourself to open and relax. Allow yourself to receive the healing energy. Silently affirm to yourself, "I am worthy of healing. I am worthy of healing. I deserve to be well." Give yourself permission to feel the ocean of love that is within you.

Breathing in. Breathing out.
Breathing in. Breathing out.
Letting go completely.
Resting.

Ending the Relaxation Period

Always come out of relaxation slowly; never jump right up. Begin by bringing your awareness back to your body. Become aware of the room around you. Without losing the feeling of quiet and calm that you have found, start to move and stretch. Take your time. Begin by gently moving your fingers and your toes. When you feel ready, gently roll to one side, with your knees bent. Rest there for a moment. Then place your hand on the floor for support and gently sit up. Whenever possible, follow the relaxation period with meditation practice.

Meditation

Meditation did not come easy for me. The first yoga class I ever took was given at Ananda Meditation Retreat in Nevada City, California. We began class with a half-hour session of postures. This was followed with some chanting and prayer to prepare us for meditation. The instructor informed us that we would sit in meditation for one hour.

I had never practiced meditation, so I was not quite sure of what to do. Everyone around me became quiet and still, with their eyes closed. I followed their example: I closed my eyes and sat there in silence. Every once in a while I opened my eyes to take a peek at what the others were doing. Everyone seemed to be in deep meditation. No one moved and no one seemed uncomfortable. They all sat there, perfectly still with their eyes closed.

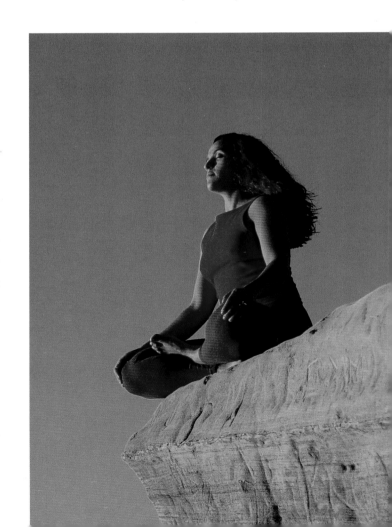

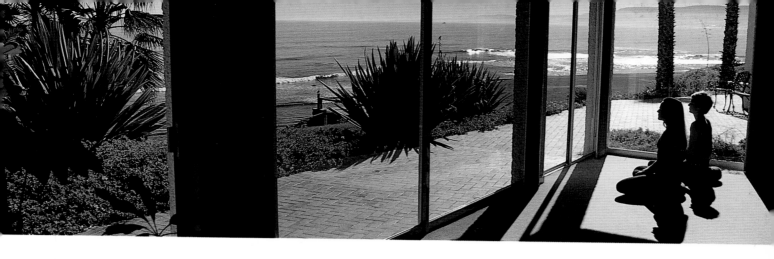

I, on the other hand, was feeling very uncomfortable. My body began to hurt from holding it upright while sitting in one position for so long. I began to notice how stiff and tight my back and neck felt. When I tried to shift my weight, my movement seemed too loud. And my mind wandered in hundreds of directions. I wanted to get up and leave the room, yet I did not want to disturb the others or call attention to myself.

When the meditation finally ended, I spoke with the instructor about my experience. I learned that during that first hour, I had not been meditating. I had not used a method to focus my mind or to quiet it. I was not even observing my thoughts. I just let them run wild and felt miserable sitting there. It was a long hour.

Meditation is a state of mind. It entails quieting the mind, emptying it, and letting go of all the chattering and racing thoughts. It is a calm, quiet state where there is no worry or confusion. When the mind is quiet, we become an open channel to higher vision, inspiration, and God consciousness. It is said that prayer is for talking to God and that meditation is for listening.

There are various methods for attaining a state of meditation. You can begin by having one point of attention to focus on, such as sitting and gazing at a candle flame or sitting with your eyes closed and repeating a word such as "peace" or "relax" silently to yourself each time you exhale. You can

also simply focus on the breath itself, feeling as it flows in and out. No matter what comes up in your mind, notice it honestly without judgment and then go back to the point of focus.

It is interesting to watch what thoughts arise from the mind. At first there are many: I feel silly sitting here, I wonder what I should have for dinner tonight, I do not like the neighbor's fence, and so on—so many thoughts. Each time I catch my mind wandering while I am meditating, I remind myself to focus again on the candle flame or on my breath or on whatever my point of focus is. It is an exercise in concentration. The process sometimes gets frustrating, but frustration is just one more thought. In time, the mind will stay quiet for longer and longer periods. Just keep bringing your attention back.

It helps to sit in a position that keeps your spine in a straight line while meditating. This keeps your energy moving upward. If you slump over or lie down, you may fall asleep. Meditation is not sleep—it is a state of relaxed alertness, a quiet awareness between the conscious and subconscious mind. Many people sit on pillows or folded blankets with their legs crossed or in a supported kneeling position. A chair is okay as long as you sit up straight, with your feet flat on the floor.

For many people, the purpose of hatha yoga is to prepare the body for sitting in meditation. It is hard to sit still for any length of time if your body

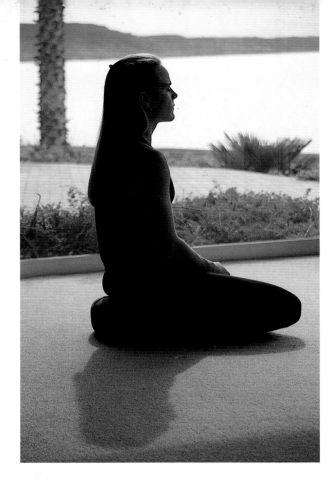

is stiff, tense, or uncomfortable. After doing postures, it is much easier to sit with the spine relaxed and erect for long periods.

Some people practice meditation even though they do not practice the postures. Of course, I recommend that you do both, but there are situations where meditation becomes the stronger ally of the two. This is true especially for those people who are bedridden, physically injured, or disabled and who are limited in their ability to move into the postures. Meditation is a practice almost anyone can engage in. It is not a passive state; it involves changing your level of consciousness and energy to a higher state of energy. Once you reach this state, you are more receptive to healing and the experience of wholeness.

Meditation happens in two stages: the getting there, which often involves using a technique, and the being there, which is the experience itself. It is a discipline that takes practice.

It is helpful to meditate in a quiet place, with the lights low but not completely dark. If finding a quiet place is difficult, try using earplugs or headphones to block out noise. If you create a specific meditation corner or meditation room in your home, you will become accustomed to relaxing your mind and body each time you sit in that area. Some people find it helpful to sit in front of an altar with candles, pictures of great saints or gurus, flowers, symbols of nature, or whatever else assists them in knowing that this is a sacred place.

Meditating outdoors in nature is also very powerful. Nature is full of prana life energy. You may have a special bench in your garden that is perfect for meditation, a favorite rock you like to sit on next to a river, or a peaceful spot under your favorite tree. Any peaceful place where you will not be interrupted is ideal. Listening to nature sounds such as birds singing, ocean waves moving in and out, or water flowing down a river can become a focus point for your meditation.

I usually meditate 10–20 minutes a day. It is enough for me, although some people sit longer. I am not always consistent; this is a weak link in my personal practice. Travel especially throws me off my meditation schedule and then I lose the value of sitting still, quieting my mind, and raising my consciousness. It is such a simple act and yet so easy to ignore.

The best way to truly reap the benefits of meditation is through daily practice. Practicing daily gives long-term results. Take, for example, brushing your teeth—you need to brush every day (or several times a day) in order to gain the benefits of healthy teeth and gums. Set aside the same time (or times) each day for your meditation so it becomes part of your routine. Ideally, meditate for 15–30 minutes at each sitting, or more if you enjoy it. But even if you only sit for 5 minutes each day, that is a great beginning, and you will notice a difference.

With regular meditation, you gain the benefits of calmness and clarity of mind, and you develop an inner awareness and receptivity to intuitive, divine guidance. On the physiological level, as you are meditating your breath and heart rates slow, you need less oxygen, and your blood pressure goes down. You enter an alpha brainwave state, which means your mind is more relaxed. Those who meditate learn to function in this relaxed physical and mental state, often carrying this over into other parts of their lives.

Many communities offer classes in meditation, and this is a good way to get started. If you are new to meditation, working with a teacher is advised. To practice meditation, try any of the following techniques.

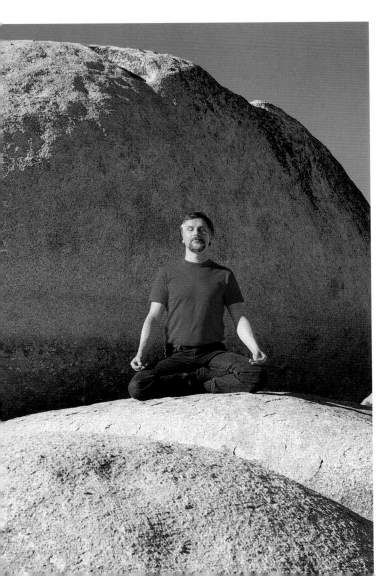

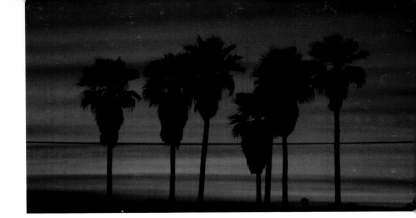

Watching Your Breath

1. Find a quiet place to sit. Observe your posture so that you are in a comfortable, upright position with your spine straight. Allow your arms to rest gently on your legs with palms facing up, or have your hands resting one over the other in your lap.

2. Close your eyes and bring your attention to your breathing. Breathe normally and observe your breath as it flows in and out of your nostrils, gently and easily.

3. Begin to notice how the temperature of your breath changes slightly at the nostrils. As the breath comes in, it is slightly cool and as the air leaves, it is slightly warm. Each time you inhale notice the coolness in your upper nostrils, and as you exhale notice that the air leaving is warmer. As you become still, you will notice your breath higher in your nose, especially at the very top of your nose.

3. Continue to stay focused on your breathing and notice that your lungs and chest expand slightly with each inhalation and then gently relax with each exhalation. You may also notice your belly moving in and out slightly. If your belly does not seem to be moving, do not worry about it. Just let your breathing flow as it wishes.

4. Do not attempt to control your breathing in any way; just observe your breathing process. Focus on the prana, the vital life-force energy entering your body with each inhalation and relaxing your body with each exhalation. If you catch your mind wandering, bring your attention back to your breathing.

5. Train your mind to become more and more aware of your breathing process. Continue to experience the alternating coolness and warmth of your breath. Continue to experience your body expanding and relaxing gently with each breath. Continue to focus on prana life energy entering and leaving your body.

6. Do this practice for as long as it is comfortable.

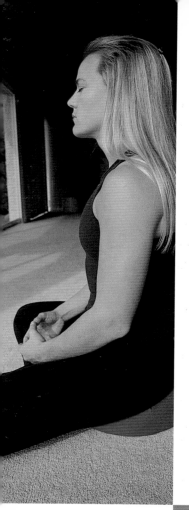

Silent Word Repetition

1. Sit in a comfortable position with your spine straight.

2. Close your eyes and begin by paying attention to your breathing. Inhale slowly and deeply. As you exhale, silently say the word "peace" slowly with the exhalation.

3. Visualize the word "peace" written in front of you. Inhale deeply, and again as you exhale silently think "peace."

4. If your mind wanders keep bringing it back to the word "peace." Keep coming back to your breathing. As your mind becomes still, your breathing continues to be slow and even.

5. Remain motionless in this position for as long as is comfortable, becoming more and more aware of what is occurring within.

Other words that can be used are love, patience, joy, calmness, light, harmony, trust, and relax.

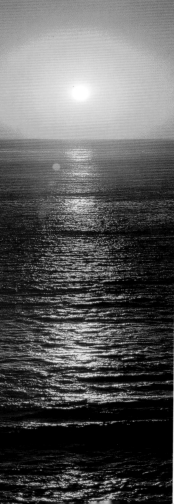

Candle Gazing: An Exercise in Concentration

1. Find a warm, quiet, dark room.

2. Place a lighted candle in the room so that you can sit and watch the flame. The candle should be at eye level about three feet away from you.

3. Gaze at the flame without blinking for a minute or two. When your eyes begin to water, close them and visualize the candle flame in your mind. As the image starts to fade, open your eyes again and gaze at the candle flame.

4. As thoughts come up in your mind, keep bringing your attention back to the candle flame.

5. If your eyes water after a short time, simply close them again and visualize the flame in your mind's eye until the image vanishes.

With practice you will gradually be able to extend the period of gazing. As your concentration goes deeper, your gaze will become steadier. In time you will be able to visualize the candle flame quite easily when you close your eyes.

Mantra Meditation

Sound is a form of energy and vibration that can have healing effects on us. The ancient yogis used mantras or Sanskrit sounds, syllables, words, and phrases that, when repeated in meditation, helped bring an individual to a higher state of consciousness. The repetition of a mantra is another way to focus your mind, and it also releases the energy that is encased in that sound. The sound vibration merges with the thought vibration; you do not need to know the meaning of the sound in order to receive its energy.

One of the most powerful Sanskrit sounds is the syllable Om.

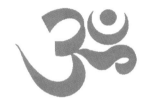

This Sanskrit word, pronounced AUM, is a mantra that has been chanted for centuries by Hindu meditators and others. It is said to be the symbolic sound of the universe, representing both the mortal and the immortal.

1. Sit in a comfortable position with your spine straight. Close your eyes.

2. To help with your concentration, begin by focusing on your breathing. Take several deep breaths and feel yourself settling into a relaxed, upright position in preparation for mantra meditation.

3. Inhale fully, and as you exhale pronounce the first long "A" sound, allowing it to generate from deep in your belly (aaaaaa). Continue sounding out, so the "A" merges into an "U" and you allow it to vibrate in your chest and heart area (oooooo). Finally, add on the "M" sound, allowing it to resonate through your entire head (mmmmm). It becomes one continuous sound, A-U-M, as you exhale. Inhale, and repeat the process. You feel both the sound and vibration as they move up through your body.

4. Chant the Om sound for several minutes. Continue the meditation by changing the Om sound to a whisper, quietly and gently on each exhalation. Complete the meditation by repeating the Om sound silently to yourself. Each time you find your mind wandering, bring it back to the mantra.

Sitting in Silence

Sometimes simply sitting in silence is healing in itself. In this practice, you bring your attention to the sounds of silence. This may include sounds of nature: the Earth, the wind, the rain, the stillness of night-time. If you are indoors, you might

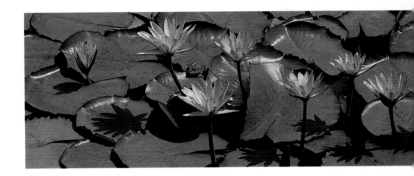

become extremely aware of a clock ticking, which you had not noticed before. Use whatever sounds you find as a focal point for your mind. Ideally, it is best to find a place and time away from activity and noise. If you live in a city, it can be helpful to spend five or ten minutes sitting in silence, perhaps in the early morning as the sun is rising or late at night when things have settled down.

Our modern world is filled with noise pollution which hinders the sounds of the natural world—traffic, television, vacuum cleaners, lawn mowers—the list goes on and on. Some people never experience the natural sounds of nature and silence. And yet silence is soothing to our nervous system. Making a conscious effort to be in silence is healing, even if it is done with earplugs.

Prayer

Prayer is a powerful practice. The moment of prayer is always an event. It is an action of recognition and honor to the invisible forces that guide our lives. As a spiritual practice, prayer works. It may work in an entirely different way than we think, and it may be that we do not recognize the answers when they come. But when we pray, answers do come.

In recent years there have been scientific studies that have demonstrated the effectiveness of prayer for health and healing. Larry Dossy, M.D., has written several books and articles about the practice of prayer in medicine. According to Dossy, experiments have shown that prayer positively affects high blood pressure, wounds, heart attacks, headaches, and anxiety. Prayer-like thoughts, offered from a distance, have been demonstrated to increase the healing rate of surgical wounds; and religious faith is associated with faster recovery from surgery. Some people think of prayer as a religious activity. Prayer can also be thought of as spiritual practice. The spirituality emphasized in *Gentle Yoga for Healing Mind, Body, Spirit* is not limited to any specific religion or denomination.

Spirituality is a universal experience that transcends race, culture, tradition, and belief. It is a feeling that emerges within us when we open our hearts to ourselves, to one another, and to the divine mystery of life. It is a feeling of connection with all living things and a feeling of wholeness that brings healing into our lives.

When I introduce prayer in my yoga classes, each student's faith is supported. Prayer is a personal practice. Through prayer we make a connection with higher reality however we may conceive of or visualize it. For some, it may be praying to God, Christ, Buddha, Mother Mary, a Great Master, or to angels and guides. Whatever faith

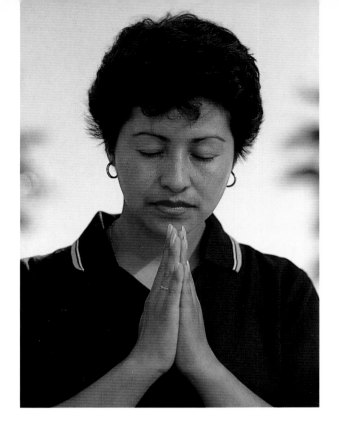

and form we choose, prayer is an offering, a giving of ourselves. Through prayer we acknowledge and express our heartfelt desire to receive guidance and protection and to send them to others. It is a life-line that links us to a higher consciousness and unites us with humanity in a spiritual way.

Loving Kindness Prayer

May I be at peace.
May my heart remain open.
May I be awakened to the light of my true nature.
May I be healed.
May I be the source of Healing for all Beings.

The Serenity Prayer

God, grant me the serenity to accept
the things I cannot change,
the courage to change the things I can,
and the wisdom to know the difference.

The Lord's Prayer

Our Father who art in heaven—
   hallowed be thy name.
Thy kingdom come, thy will be done,
On Earth as it is in heaven.
Give us this day our daily bread;
   and forgive us our debt
As we forgive our debtors.
And lead us not into temptation,
   but deliver us from evil.
For thine is the kingdom, and the power,
   and the glory
forever and ever.
Amen.

Prayer of St. Francis

Lord, make me an instrument of thy peace:
where there is hatred—let me sow Love;
where there is injury—Pardon;
where there is doubt—Faith;
where there is despair—Hope;
where there is darkness—Light;
where there is sadness—Joy.
O divine Master,
grant that I may not so much seek to be consoled,
   as to console;
to be understood, as to understand;
to be loved, as to love.
For it is in giving that we receive;
it is in pardoning that we are pardoned;
it is in dying that we are born to eternal Life.

Seneca Prayer

Oh, Great Mystery—
Grant that I walk
A path with heart
Forever in balance and harmony.

Sioux Prayer

Grandfather, great Spirit
fill us with the Light;
give us the strength to understand
and the eyes to see.
Teach us to walk the soft Earth
   as relatives to all that live.

Sufi Invocation

Toward the One
The perfection of love, harmony, and beauty.
The only being.
United with all the illuminated souls
Who form the embodiment of the Master
The spirit of guidance.

Prayer of Compassion

May all beings be free from suffering.
May all beings be at peace.
Peace, Shanti, Shanti, Peace.
May all beings be healed.

Psalm 116

I love the Lord because He hears my prayers
   and answers them.
Because He bends down and listens,
   I will pray as long as I breathe.
Thy will be done.

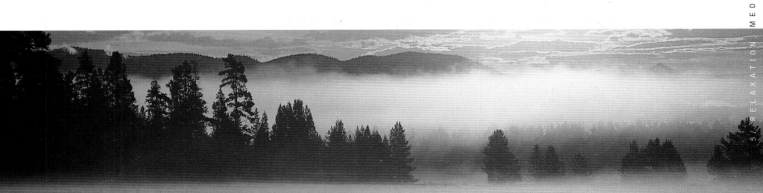

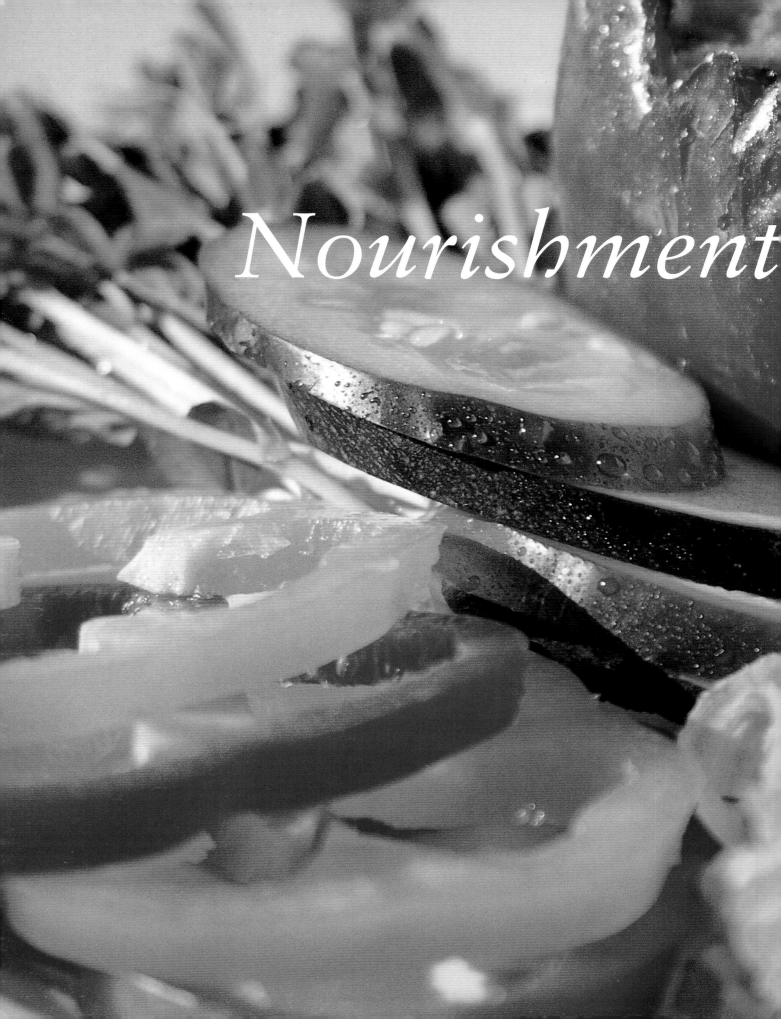

Nourishment

with Food

When I began studying hatha yoga, I was introduced to the idea of eating food to improve health and vitality. I learned that some foods give me more energy and others actually deplete my energy. I was in my early twenties at the time and was very self-conscious about my weight. There is a great amount of pressure in our culture to look and stay thin. I remember thinking of food in terms of calories and weight loss rather than vitamins, minerals, and enzymes that nourish me. I tried various diets, always vowing to lose weight and always failing. I was perhaps 5–8 pounds heavier than my ideal weight, but my desire to be thinner was on my mind all the time.

Yoga taught me to view food in a different way. I learned which foods help heal the body and which foods have a negative effect and place stress on the system. Because I was also learning to reduce stress through stretching, breathing, and relaxation, I did not have an urge to eat when I was not hungry. As my body became healthier, I began to actually crave the foods that were healthy for me; nonnutritious filler foods were no longer appealing. Without trying, I began to lose weight. I also began to have more energy and vitality.

Most yogis advocate a vegetarian diet of pure, fresh, natural foods. The closer a food is to its natural state—fresh, unfrozen, unprocessed, and unrefined—the better it is for you. Just as prana life energy is in the air we breathe, it is also in the food we eat. Food that is high in prana is fresh, pure, natural, nutritional food. The yogic way of eating is natural and compassionate. Yoga offers diet recommendations that are designed to keep our bodies functioning at their best, give us the most energy, and contain the fewest toxins.

These guidelines also adhere to the yogic principle of ahisma or nonviolence. Eating meat is discouraged to prevent the unnecessary killing of animals. Nonviolence toward fellow beings is extended to include not injuring the environment,

97

in order to protect the planet. Eating foods that have been sprayed with chemicals and pesticides is a form of injury to the environment and to our own bodies as we ingest these toxins.

As you read through this chapter, I ask you to keep an open mind. The dietary changes I advocate do not have to be made all at once. Gradual changes are often more permanent than those that happen overnight. Also, each person is unique. People with specific food allergies need to adjust their diet choices to their body chemistry and condition. Diet is a very individual matter, yet all of us can bring conscious awareness to improve our eating habits. This is one more way to nurture ourselves and enhance health. Eating nutritious foods can help reduce stress and allow the body to repair and strengthen its natural defenses against disease. With healthy eating habits, we gain more energy, vitality, strength, and endurance.

Fast Food Is Dead Food

One of the first rules of nutrition I learned when I began studying hatha yoga was: "Do not eat dead foods." At first, I did not know what that meant. I had never thought about food as being alive; I certainly had not thought that some foods had more life than others. Then it was pointed out to me that foods with life energy are the foods that give life energy to me—they give me the nutrients my body needs.

Dead foods are those foods that have been robbed of their natural vitamins, minerals, amino acids, and enzymes due to processing. They include canned, preserved, bleached, polished, refined, and otherwise devitalized foods.

Oftentimes these dead foods are presented to us as fast foods and convenience foods. They are called convenient because they are easy to prepare and they save us time. Just open a can or take a package out of the freezer, heat it up and in 10 minutes you have a meal. If you have not eaten at home, you can always grab a quick bite to eat at a nearby fast-food restaurant. Television commercials advertise the fun and convenience of ordering a pizza or enjoying a burger and fries with our loved ones. The advertisements do not mention the nutritional value of such food, perhaps because there is none. Fast foods are generally refined; high in fat, sugar, and salt and nutrient-poor. Although they may work just fine to soothe your appetite, they do little to give you the necessary vitamins, minerals, amino acids, and enzymes that your body needs—and to build and maintain a healthy body.

Foods for Reducing Stress and Building Health

Fruits and Vegetables

Eat lots of fresh fruits and vegetables. Make a big green salad with a variety of raw vegetables as part of your daily diet—it is excellent for your health. Raw vegetables contain plenty of nutrients and fiber that your body needs. Cooked vegetables are also fine as long as they are not overcooked, so that all the vitamins and minerals are lost. Ask for lightly steamed vegetables whenever possible.

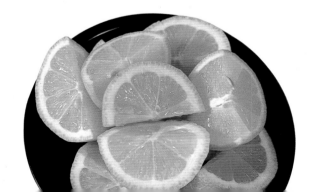

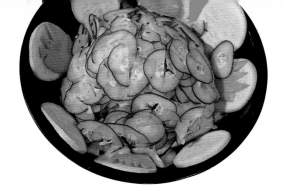

Baked carrots, squash, and potatoes are also very good; it is what we put on top of them that hurts us: sugar, butter, and sour cream. Sea vegetables such as kelp, nori, and kombo are excellent mineral sources and taste great when added to soups. They can usually be found in health food stores.

Avoid canned fruits and vegetables because these are often dead foods that contain added sugar and salt.

Vegetable Juices

Fresh vegetable juices are a good source of enzymes, minerals, and other nutrients. Buying a juicer is a worthwhile investment. You can have juice several times a day, as a between-meal snack or with a meal. For best results, consume the juice within 15 minutes of juicing the vegetables. Because carrot juice can raise your blood sugar, dilute it in half with green vegetable juice or water.

Organic Produce: Is It Worth It?

Organically grown foods are those produced without chemical fertilizers or pesticides. Most farms are required to farm organically for three years before the food they produce can be labeled "certified organic." This allows time for the soil to be remineralized and for harmful chemicals to be removed. The popularity of organic produce is growing rapidly as people begin to recognize the harmful effects of the huge amounts of pesticides sprayed on farmland each year. The consumption of organic products can reduce the risks of chemical exposure, both to individuals and to the planet. Organic foods are not only free of chemical

residue, but they taste better and have many more nutrients than commercially farmed foods.

To help improve your health and the health of the environment buy organic, local, and seasonal produce whenever possible. The more we support organic farmers, the less pesticides are produced. I have heard some people complain that organic food is more expensive and that they cannot afford the extra cost. I say you cannot afford not to make sure you are eating nontoxic foods. You are worth the extra cost—it is an investment in your health and your planet.

Whole Grains and Legumes

Gradually reduce and eliminate refined foods from your diet. These include white sugar, white flour, white bread, white rice, and white pasta products. Eat whole grains instead. Look for products such as whole-wheat or rye flour, multi-grain breads and cereals, brown rice, oats, millet, and buckwheat. Once you make up your mind to stop eating refined foods, you will find lots of options available. You may have to adjust at first to new textures and tastes, but remember that refined foods have been stripped of important nutrients and fiber. Even though they taste good, they place more stress on your system.

Whole grains are rich in B-complex vitamins, which play an essential role in keeping stress levels down. Whole grains also supply important amino acids to the body, especially when eaten with legumes. Combinations such as beans and rice or rice and lentil soap make great meals.

Nuts and Seeds

Nuts and seeds are healthy snack foods, especially if eaten raw. These foods are good sources of protein, but are also high in oils, so if you are on a fat-restricted diet you will need to limit your intake. Avoid roasted nuts that have been heavily salted.

Adding nuts and seeds to your meals is fun and nutritious. Unhulled sesame seeds are high in calcium and taste delicious when sprinkled on grains. Sunflower seeds, pumpkin seeds, and almonds are great in salads or eaten alone.

I like to take a handful of almonds with me in my pocket when I know I will be having a busy day and will need extra energy. If I am working long hours and cannot take the time to have a complete meal, I can eat a few almonds throughout my day to keep my blood sugar from dropping. This is really important because low-blood-sugar cravings often result in binging and overeating.

Water

Water is one of the essential compounds in our body chemistry. An insufficient intake of water is often responsible for constipation, liver and kidney malfunctions, congested colon, and poor cell functioning. The only way to allow the body's sophisticated filtration system to work properly is to take in enough water to flush out the toxins that build up.

You should drink at least six 8-oz. glasses of water every day. This is in addition to whatever other beverages you drink. Pure water helps your body excrete toxins. Water also regulates your body temperature and transports nutrients throughout your system.

It is best to drink purified, spring, or distilled water. This is preferable to the processed, softened, or polluted tap water that is found in many communities.

Foods to Consider Reducing from Your Diet

Dairy Products

For years I ate dairy products as one of my main foods. I especially liked cheese. I also drank milk and used it on my cereals. In my early thirties, I developed allergies to various pollens and molds in the air. A friend suggested that if I stopped eating dairy products my allergies would get better because dairy products create mucus in the system. Because I was miserable, I tried following my friend's advice—and my allergies cleared up. You may want to try this experiment yourself.

Since that time I have eaten very little dairy. In place of milk, I use soy milk, which tastes great to me. I seldom eat cheese. If I do eat cheese, I make sure it is natural and not processed with added sugar, salt, and preservatives. Always read the labels. Soy cheeses are also available, although I have to admit that they do not taste good to me. However, I have friends who like soy cheese. You have to experiment for yourself.

Use butter in very small amounts. Butter is made from cream and is high in saturated fats. Keeping fat out of your diet reduces the risk of heart disease. Butter is better than margarine because margarine contains artificial additives and preservatives. Health food stores sell natural oil spreads that can be substituted for butter. Ghee is another product found in health food stores that is a healthy replacement for butter.

Yogurt is a good source of protein and contains friendly bacteria that aid in digestion and intestinal functions. Look for natural yogurt that does not contain added sugar and artificial flavorings.

Eggs

Everyone knows that eggs are a good source of protein. Years ago I raised my own chickens and

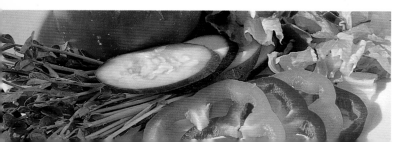

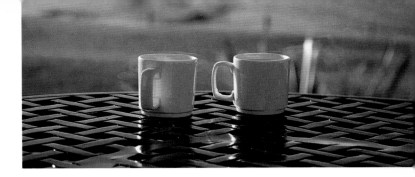

discovered the difference between fresh eggs and store-bought eggs. Fresh eggs definitely taste better. Although I seldom eat eggs these days, when I do I look for fresh brown eggs. Health food stores usually carry them and get them locally. It is best to eat eggs that have been poached or boiled rather than fried in oil or scrambled in butter. Fried foods of any kind are hard on the digestive system. Eggs are high in cholesterol and should be avoided if that is a concern. Tofu can be used as an egg replacement for scrambled eggs (see the recipe at the end of the chapter).

Meat

There was a time when cows, pigs, sheep, chickens, and turkeys were raised organically on farms. They had healthy, natural lives. But these days the meat and poultry industries keep these animals locked up in crowded factories where they are severely mistreated and stuffed with chemicals, steroids, and antibiotics. After they are slaughtered, they are prepared with more additives and preservatives for our markets.

Because of this, many people avoid eating meat completely. If you choose to eat meat, look for meat that has been organically grown and is not filled with additives and preservatives. Processed meat such as bacon, ham, cold cuts, hot dogs, salami, and sausages contain numerous additives and are usually processed with some kind of sugar as a preservative. Read labels. Red meats such as beef and pork are high in saturated fat. Poultry and fish tend to be lower in saturated fats than other meats.

I cannot help thinking that spiritually we pay a price when we eat animals that have been kept in pain and terror throughout their lives. The grain that is used to feed and fatten livestock could feed five times the U.S. population. Hunger and malnutrition could be alleviated worldwide if we used that grain to feed people. Whether or not you agree with this view, it does merit some thought.

Sugar and caffeine

Sugar and caffeine offer no nutritional value for our bodies. In small amounts they may do no harm, if you are healthy. If your health is compromised, these substances will add additional stress to your system. Sugar and caffeine lower our bodies' ability to fight stress and to heal. Caffeine actually draws B vitamins out of the body. Both of these substances can be addictive, and that of course is part of the problem.

If you have a weakness for sugar or caffeine then pay attention to your energy levels. Observe how these substances affect your overall feeling of well being. When you first eat sugar or drink caffeine your blood sugars will rise quickly, stimulating your energy. But after a short while your blood sugars fall and you feel tired, often craving more sugar or caffeine. To avoid this up and down addictive cycle we need to eat healthy food in healthy amounts, which will keep our blood sugars stable.

Stopping or reducing your intake of sugar and caffeine is not always easy, especially if you have become addicted. You may experience some withdrawal symptoms if you quit cold turkey. Read labels and notice how many foods contain these substances. If you don't feel ready or willing to give up sugar or caffeine completely, then work on reducing your intake.

I suggest that you start by replacing sugar with fresh fruit. Whenever you get a craving for something sweet try eating an apple. Apples are easy to take along with you wherever you go. At first you may feel deprived of those sweets you love but your mind will soon adapt as you become calmer, clearer, and healthier. When this happens your cravings for sugar will decrease.

As for caffeine, there are plenty of decaffeinated coffees and beverages available. I struggle with this addiction myself. I often start my day with a cup of coffee. I enjoy the flavor. I like the lift that coffee gives me, and when I travel I enjoy buying specialty coffees to bring home with me. Caffeine is a very popular drug worldwide, perhaps the most popular. Although I have a habit of drinking coffee, I limit my intake. And I pay attention to my energy levels. If I am sick or feeling fatigued and stressed, I stop drinking coffee completely until I feel better again. I want to give my body all the energy it needs for healing.

Each time I quit drinking coffee I feel sluggish for a few days as the caffeine is leaving my system, but afterwards I feel renewed energy and calmness of mind. My energy is stable rather than stimulated. I have gone without coffee for months at a time. So far I have always returned to the habit. Perhaps one day I will quit forever.

If your health is compromised in any way then I suggest you eliminate sugar and caffeine from your diet. You may be surprised at how much more energy you have for healing, once you get through the initial withdrawal from cravings. If you need medical support while quitting these substances, I suggest you find a nutritional doctor in your local area. Nutritional medicine is a specialty in and of itself, with many excellent practitioners who can guide you.

General Rules for Eating

- Eat slowly. Chew your food thoroughly. Digestion begins in the mouth.

- Allow time for your food to digest. Eating your meals in a relaxing environment without external distractions enhances your body's ability to digest and assimilate food effectively. Often people eat on the run; it is common to see people gulping down food as they rush off to

FOODS TO REDUCE OR ELIMINATE

- Sugars and sweets: candy, ice cream, sugar-sweetened drinks, sugar-filled desserts, sugar coated cereals, and so on

- Caffeine: coffee, tea, cola, cocoa, and chocolates

- Refined foods (foods that contain additives and preservatives): sausages, bacon, cold cuts, hot dogs, salami, and so on

- Salt (causes fluid retention, high blood pressure, and heart disease)

- Canned foods (contain added sugar and salt)

- Condiments: mayonnaise, ketchup, pickles, and rich salad dressing (contain added sugar and salt)

- Meat and dairy products: look for organic and farm-raised—if you can eat these.

ADD AND ENJOY

- Fresh fruits and vegetables (should make up 50–70% of your diet)

- Whole grains: brown rice, oats, millet, buckwheat, multigrain breads, and so on

- Legumes: peas, lentils, and beans

- Nuts and seeds (best eaten raw, unsalted, and in small quantities)

- Soy milk products (can replace dairy products)

- Fresh white fish (can replace meat)

- Herbal teas: peppermint, apple cinnamon, chamomile, and so on

- Water (at least six 8-oz. glasses a day)

work. This does not make for good digestion. Nurture yourself by enjoying sit-down meals eaten in a calm environment. Take your time.

- Drink 6–8 glasses of pure water daily. It is best to drink fluids between your meals.

- If you snack, choose healthy foods. Keep an assortment of healthy snack foods readily available in case you feel hungry. Celery sticks, an apple, or a bag of almonds are examples of healthy snack choices that will help curb your appetite and give you the added benefit of proper nutrition.

- Make a habit of reading the labels on foods. Avoid foods with additives, preservatives, and sugars.

A Few Recipes to Get Started

In the bibliography, you will find recommended cookbooks that follow some of the healthy eating guidelines I have recommended. Here I provide just a few recipes to get you started. Exploring new ways of preparing healthy meals is a fun project. Bon apetit!

SCRAMBLED TOFU

> 1 pound firm tofu
> ½ teaspoon vegetable oil
> 1 small onion, diced
> ½ cup mushrooms, sliced
> ½ cup green bell peppers, diced
> 1 clove garlic, minced
> ½ teaspoon thyme
> ½ teaspoon curry powder
> 1 tablespoon tamari
> ½ teaspoon sea salt
> a pinch of black pepper
> ¼ cup water

In a small mixing bowl, cut and crumble the tofu with a fork. In a skillet, heat the oil and sauté the onions, mushrooms, and green peppers. Stir in the tofu, seasonings, and water. Cook over low heat 3–5 minutes. Adjust seasonings to taste. Serve and enjoy.

RED POTATOES WITH HERBS AND GARLIC

> 6 small red potatoes
> 2 tablespoons chopped fresh herbs (rosemary, basil, and parsley)
> ½ red onion, diced
> 2 cloves of garlic, diced
> 1 teaspoon salt
> 1 teaspoon pepper
> ¼ cup olive oil

Cook the potatoes in a pan in boiling water until they are soft but not falling apart. In a frying pan, heat the oil and sauté the onion and garlic. Add the herbs, sea salt, pepper, and potatoes; sauté until potatoes are lightly browned. Serve and enjoy.

MISO SOUP

> 2 teaspoons vegetable oil
> 2 teaspoons fresh ginger, grated
> several finely chopped/sliced vegetables (cabbage, celery, carrots, potatoes, kale)
> 1 tablespoon dried wakame seaweed
> 4 cups water
> 4 tablespoons light miso
> 2 tablespoons parsley, finely chopped

In a frying pan, heat the oil and sauté the ginger and vegetables for about 5 minutes. Meanwhile, soak the wakame seaweed 4–6 minutes and then chop it. In a soup pan, place the water, chopped wakame, and vegetables. Cover and bring the mixture to a boil; reduce heat and simmer 15 minutes. Cream the miso with some of the broth, and then stir the miso-broth mixture into the soup and remove the pan from the heat. Serve immediately garnished with parsley.

BROWN RICE WITH VEGETABLES

1 cup brown rice

2 tablespoons sunflower oil

1/4 cup onion, chopped

2 cloves garlic

1 tablespoon fresh ginger, chopped

Braggs liquid aminos to taste (an all purpose seasoning made from soy protein—sold in most health food stores)

2 cups water

1/2 cup carrots, diced

1/2 cup celery, chopped

1/2 cup zucchini, diced

In a frying pan, brown rice briefly in oil until brown. In a blender, combine the onion, garlic, ginger, and tamari and blend until liquid. In a cooking pan, add the water to the rice and then add the contents of the blender. Cook over low heat, covered, for 30 minutes. After 30 minutes, add the carrots, celery, and zucchini and cook another 10 minutes, covered. Remove the pan from heat, let stand 5 minutes, and then serve.

SIMPLE AND HEALTHY SALAD DRESSING

1/4 cup olive oil

1/4 cup lemon juice

1 teaspoon tamari or sea salt

1 tablespoon freshly chopped herbs (your choice)

Put all ingredients in a screw-top jar and shake them up to combine them into dressing. Pour over a green salad (preferably made with fresh organic vegetables). Makes 1/2 cup.

APPLE SAUCE

This is a tasty dessert.

10 apples, cored and diced

3/4 cup water or pure apple juice

1 lemon, juiced

cinnamon and nutmeg to taste

Put the diced apples and water or apple juice into a large pan. Bring this to a boil, reduce heat, and simmer until the apples are soft. Add the lemon juice and spices. Serve warm or chilled. Makes 6–8 cups.

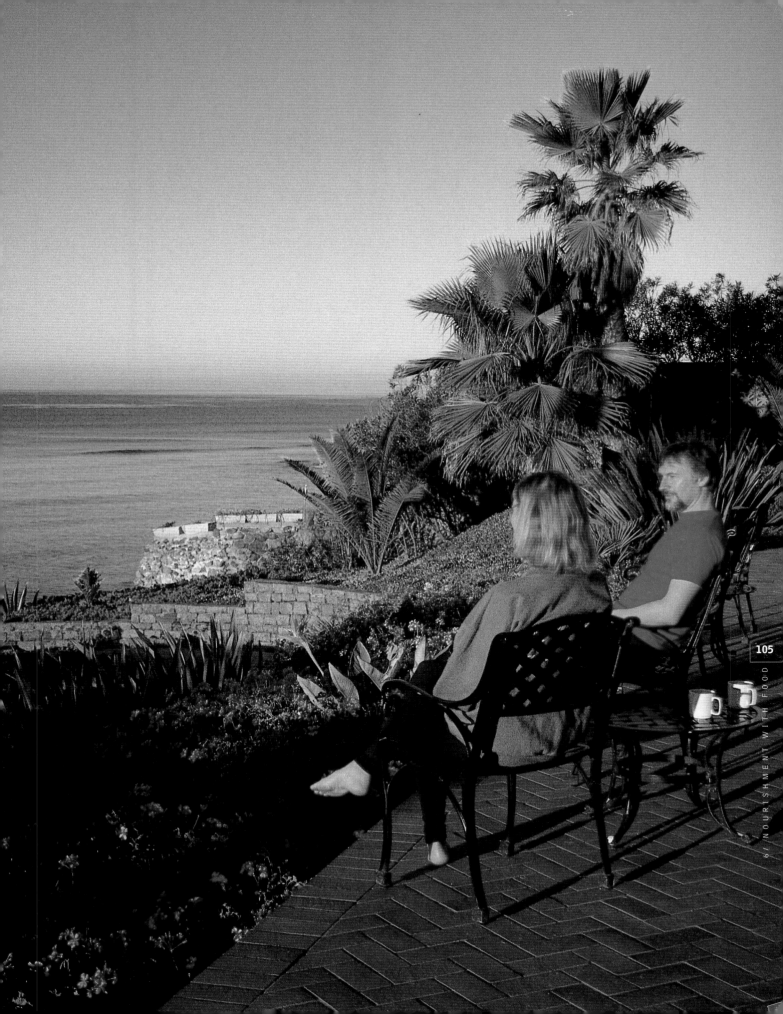

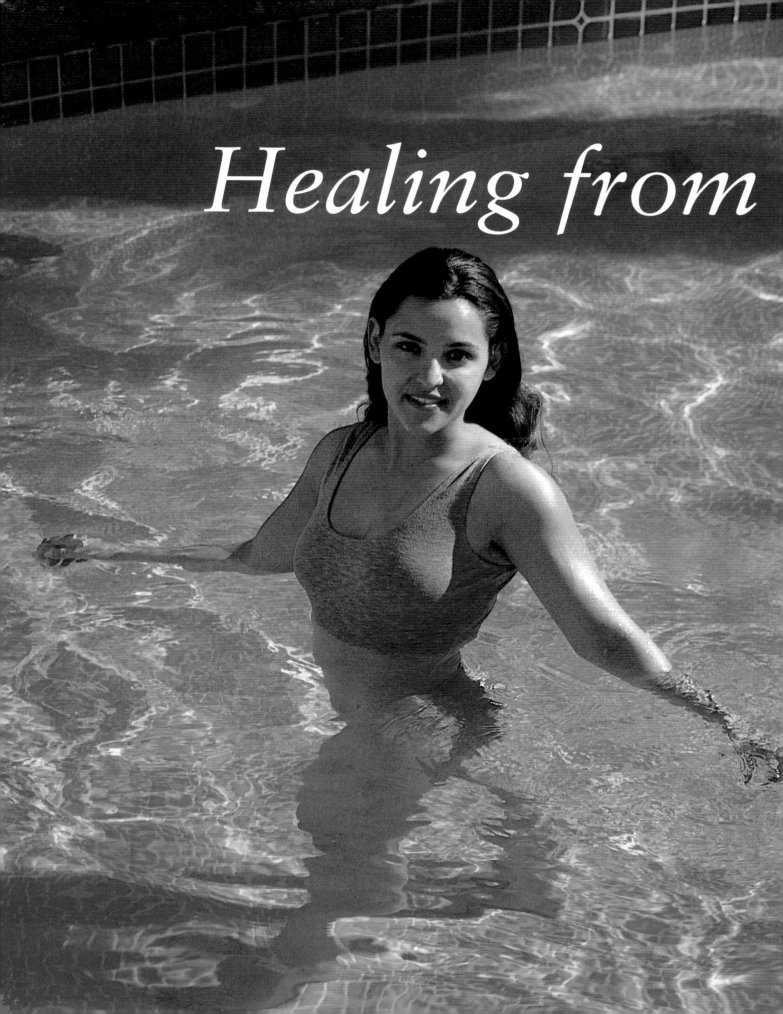

Healing from

CHAPTER SEVEN

Injury and Illness

I am not a medical expert. I always recommend that people who have illnesses or injuries seek medical advice before attending my yoga class. I welcome these people to the classes with an understanding and agreement from them that we will be very cautious and respectful of their bodies' natural healing processes. Patience is always encouraged. Sometimes people come to class and stay in relaxation pose the entire time. Even if people are unable to participate fully in the yoga practices, they can still benefit from the positive affirmations, visualizations, and relaxation exercises and from being with a group of warm, caring people in an uplifting environment.

It has been wonderful to see improvements in people's lives as a result of yoga practices and teachings. I have had numerous experiences in working with people with injuries or illnesses who credit yoga practice as a major contributor to their healing process. I have also worked with my own injuries from a car accident and with health challenges from allergies. I view gentle yoga practice as

a wonderful adjunct to healing. In most medical situations, there will be a place for both suggested medical treatments and gentle yoga practices such as breath work, simple adaptive movements, massage, relaxation, meditation, and prayer.

Again, I emphasize that it is important to consult your doctor or medical adviser before beginning yoga practice if you are sick or injured. Take things very slowly. If you pay attention to your energy level and the discomfort signals of your body, you will know when you have done enough and need to rest. Sometimes rest is all that is required. The guided relaxation period during yoga class can assist in promoting deep rest. Visualization practice can assist in pain management. Breathing exercises can assist in bringing more prana (healing life energy) to areas that need healing. There are many ways to benefit from gentle simple practices.

One of the benefits of practicing gentle yoga techniques during a health crisis is that it gives you a vehicle to actively participate in your own healing process. When we become engaged in our own healing process, we feel less helpless and more empowered to create change. An optimistic attitude can enhance our immune function, but a helpless or hopeless attitude may depress immune function. Even if our greatest healing is simply to find peace of mind and acceptance of our condition, engaging in that process is positive.

The Mind-Body Connection

The mind-body connection has to do with understanding that the mind and body are not separate, that they have always been together, and that they have an interactive influence on one another. Mind-body medicine has gained tremendous acceptance in the past decade. Numerous studies have been done to demonstrate that our thoughts and emotions do indeed affect our health and well-being. In addition, the influences of diet has been included in some studies, along with the influence of belief in faith and spirituality.

There are several names to describe this field of study: mind-body medicine, attitudinal healing, and psychoneuroimmunology (PNI). PNI is an area of scientific research that explores the relationship between mind, emotions, and body. It has found, for instance, that when we laugh our bodies produce healing chemicals that enhance the immune function and reduce pain. Numerous excellent books have been written about the mind-body connection by experts such as Herbert Benson, Joan Borysenkop, Deepak Chopra, Larry Dossey, Christine Northrup, Dean Ornish, Norman Shealy, Bernie Siegel, Andrew Weil, and others (see the bibliography).

As someone who has been practicing yoga for over 20 years, I am so pleased to find scientific data that validates ancient yogic teachings. I say

this because many people seem to be more convinced about the practical benefits of addressing mind-body health because scientific data has demonstrated that these benefits are possible; they are now more likely to believe me when I say things like: "Our thoughts have energy. Our minds can positively influence our physiology and health. Laughter stimulates the immune system. What we eat affects how we feel. Our emotions affect our health. Relaxation is a skill that anyone can learn."

Ancient yoga wisdom has always considered our well-being as an integrated whole. All aspects of health are acknowledged. Hatha yoga focuses on the health and wellness of the physical body, balance and integration of the mind and emotions, and the awakening of the spiritual dimension of being.

We humans are physical, mental-emotional, and spiritual beings. These different aspects of ourselves are affected by one another. For example, our thoughts and emotions have physiological effects on us: When we are embarrassed, we blush; when we are nervous, our heart rates increase and our palms may sweat; and when we find something boring, we may yawn.

If a situation makes me feel bad emotionally, then I have less energy physically. Any physical pain will disturb my mental outlook on life. When I am in touch with my spirituality, I feel better emotionally. When I feel good physically, it is easier to meditate, which helps me get in touch with my spiritual self. All these aspects are interrelated. If we ignore any one aspect, the rest suffer.

Stress and Illness

Most doctors now agree that stress contributes to illness. A key element in understanding the relationship between illness and the mind-body paradigm is the relationship between illness and stress.

Stress taxes our immune systems. It does so by keeping us in the fight-or-flight response.

The fight-or-flight response is a natural response. When we feel threatened, our bodies react by shifting into high gear, into overdrive, in order to survive the real or imagined threat. When this happens, our bodies secrete a variety of hormones, including adrenaline and cortisol. These hormones affect our health in various ways. On the one hand, they give us energy and strength. You may have heard the story of the woman whose child was trapped under a 110-ton truck. Without pausing to think, she ran over to the truck, lifted it up, and released her child. It is okay to have a fight-or-flight response now and then.

On the other hand, when we become caught in a chronic state of fight-or-flight alertness, we get in trouble. Our nervous system keeps cycling in high gear and our immune system suffers. Our breathing becomes rapid so it can deliver a rush of oxygen to our muscles. Our muscles become tense. As adrenaline pours out of our adrenal glands, our blood pressure rises and our heart beats more forcefully. Sugar is released from the liver into the bloodstream. At the same time our digestive system and kidneys shut down; these systems are put on hold until the threat passes.

Unfortunately, if we continue to perceive the world as dangerous and stressful, the threat never passes. The key word here is "perceive." Our bodies respond to what is happening in our minds as if it were real. Any perception of physical or emotional threat can trigger the fight-or-flight response. And it can become a vicious cycle. The more often we view the world as stressful, the more often the body goes into the fight-or-flight response. Chronic stress taxes our immune system. Over time, our health is compromised which in turn, gives us more stress.

Through yoga we learn to step out of this state of chronic stress and move in the direction of wholeness, physical health, and spiritual consciousness. The methods used in hatha yoga are congruent with mind-body medicine. They work to improve physical health and well-being, increase mental concentration and clarity, balance and calm the emotions, and, through meditation, enable us to come closer to the realization of our own spiritual nature. With these tools, stress becomes more manageable, and perceptions change.

Igniting the Healer Within

Our lives are so busy these days. With all the gifts that technology has given us, it has taken its toll on our bodies. Sitting for long periods of time, driving, talking on cell phones, and living at a fast pace create stress. Many of us have forgotten what it feels like to be deeply relaxed. We forget that we are connected to nature and her power to nourish us, heal us and restore our energy. Our ability to focus on healing energy often remains hidden during our busy, activity-filled days.

Yoga teaches that every action and thought we have is either enhancing our life energy or dissipating it. When we consciously choose activities and thoughts that enhance our life energy, we support our bodies' natural ability to heal. The stronger and more vibrant our life energy is, the better we feel. When we are sick or injured, this becomes even more important—our energy is weakened and it requires extra care. Deep attention is needed for healing and renewal of our bodies and souls.

When people are sick or in pain they often rely on medications. After experiencing tremendous physical pain as a result of being in a car accident, I was grateful to have pain medication and anti-inflammatories available to me. There is a time and a place for using medication. But it is also important to embrace lifestyle choices that enhance our bodies' natural ability to heal our condition. In this culture, which is focused on productivity and consumerism, we have a tendency to ignore our inner selves. When we get sick or injured, we look for something outside to fix us. People who experience stress symptoms such as anxiety, headaches, ulcers, or insomnia often rely on tranquilizers, aspirin, antacids, or other medications to get them through the day.

A healthier way to deal with such symptoms is to focus your awareness on awakening your body's natural ability to heal. We have an innate healing wisdom within us, sometimes known as intuition or inner-knowing. Accessing it and allowing it to guide us is the challenging part. It takes time and commitment to hear our inner guide tell us what will nurture us. When we relax the body and mind, the greater knowledge from within comes to the surface. Some people have received profound messages about themselves and their healing process from quieting their being and listening within. You can become an ally to your body by treating symptoms of illness as messages telling you to slow down, eat healthier foods, rest, play, relax, and nurture yourself. Learning to become engaged in our own healing process is possible and empowering.

The last time I was in Hawaii, I slipped on some coral and cut my leg. The wound was pretty deep. I went back to the home I was staying in and immediately put some ice on the swelling and antibacterial cream on the cut. I also placed my hands over the wound and imagined that I was sending healing energy into the leg. The next day, the wound looked worse. I could have been worried, but instead I put faith in my body's healing process. My body's own natural intelligence knows how to heal wounds. There were a few days when the wound looked nasty. It turned white, sur-

rounded by red. Each night I kept imagining the wound as healed. By using this imagery, I was supporting my body's natural ability to heal with positive energy. The good news is that it never got infected and within two weeks it had completely healed.

Our bodies have a healing power. Each time we cut ourselves, the cut heals. It may take a week or two. It may require our assistance in keeping it clean and protected. But all the while, the body's innate healing capabilities are at work healing the cut. If we sprain our ankle, the sprain will eventually heal. Each time we catch a cold or come down with the flu, the body moves into a mode of healing. Healing is a natural, innate process. We can either pay attention to the messages that are asking us to take greater care of ourselves or we can ignore those messages and work against our bodies' attempt to heal the condition. The choice is ours. Our consciousness also has a healing power. If we become engaged in our own healing process, we demonstrate our respect for the subtle energies of the body and mind, which reveal the secrets of balance, harmony, and the release of energy for healing. In essence we allow for greater healing with our active cooperation and support in the process.

Sometimes, in spite of their best efforts people still remain sick, and sometimes people die. Life can appear to be quite unjust. Yoga embraces the philosophy that we are whole beings. When we are ill, we are more than our disease. We are more than our symptoms. Healing comes from the root "to make whole." Although curing is not always possible in every situation, the transformation of true healing is. When we find peace, we experience our wholeness. I have always found this to be a comforting thought.

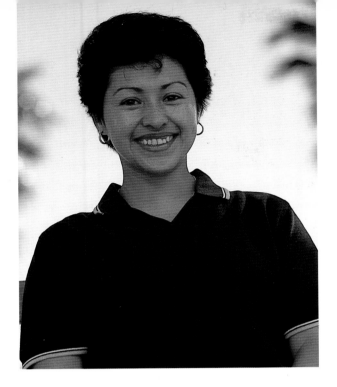

Focused Attention on Healing

The more attention we place on something, the greater influence it has in our lives. If we focus on the discomfort and pain in our body, it will consume us. If we focus on healing our body, mind, and emotions, we will see transformations in these aspects of our lives.

When we experience discomfort or pain from injury or illness we can use our attention to direct a healing response to the area that requires our care. Focusing our attention on a part of our body with the intention of bringing healing energy to that area will have a different effect than focusing on the expectation of pain. We become part of the solution rather than identifying with the problem. Visualization is a powerful way to mobilize the inner healer with our focused attention. Our mind and body cooperate together to allow for relaxation and receptivity to healing.

People experience pain in different ways. You may feel pain as tightness, contraction, throbbing sensations, heat, constriction, or dull aching. Pain has a definite way of getting our attention. When pain or sickness grabs our attention, we need to meet it in a positive loving way. It is easy to get discouraged when you do not feel well. Use your mind for healing instead. Imagine yourself getting well. Picture yourself enjoying activities that you love. Focus your awareness on simple pleasures: the warmth of your favorite blanket, the sound of soothing music, fresh flowers next to your bed.

When using imagery for healing it's important to stay relaxed, focused, and directed. Some people like to work with images of melting and releasing the pain. You might use images such as snow or butter melting. Or see the area flooded with light, helping it to melt and release. You can also use visualization to focus on what your body felt like before you were sick or injured. In this way visualization is used to reawaken the memory of health.

If you have an injury or illness, you may want to study basic anatomy and the specific elements of your treatment process to help visualize the best results. Take time each day to imagine yourself as a healthy person. See yourself in an environment that you love.

RELAXATION VISUALIZATION FOR PAIN MANAGEMENT

1. Lie down in a comfortable position. Close your eyes. Breathe deeply. Slowly exhale, allowing the tension in your chest, shoulders, and abdomen to release. Continue taking deep full breaths and allow each exhalation to take you to a quieter, more comfortable, more relaxed state of being.

2. Bring your awareness to the place of discomfort or pain that calls for your attention. There is no need to resist the sensation; rather, bring your attention to your breathing as you allow the muscles in your neck, shoulders, arms, and legs to relax.

3. Continue taking deep breaths and allow your body to release tension with every exhalation. Feel the area of pain or discomfort relaxing gradually, slowly letting go as you continue breathing and relaxing all other parts of your body. Your teeth are slightly parted so that your jaw is relaxed. Your face is relaxed. Your arms and legs are relaxed. Your body sinks heavier into the floor beneath you. You feel the holding and tightness in your body letting go. Continue breathing and letting go.

4. Imagine that you are lying down on a blanket on top of soft grass or on a warm sandy beach. The air is warm, the sun is shining, the sky is clear, and everything around you is beautiful and serene. Feel the soothing sun shining down on your body. Enjoy this time of peace and serenity. You are in a beautiful and safe place. Continue breathing and letting go. Now envision your own body as a cocoon of healing energy. Visualize and feel the life force radiating within and around you. With every breath you take, you activate this life energy. Notice any area in your body that is not well and visualize a warm, healing light surrounding that area. You are relaxed and receptive to healing. This warm soothing light fills your entire being and helps bring comfort to any area of illness or injury. All holding and tightness of pain melt away. Allow this warm, healing light to radiate comfort, peace, and love throughout your body, encompassing every cell. You are relaxed and receptive to healing.

5. Stay here as long as you need to. Allow the nourishing energy of the environment—the pure air, the nurturing earth, the luminous sun—to infuse your entire being, purifying and nourishing your body, mind, and soul. Rest with the awareness that a healing force is surrounding you. Your natural recuperative powers are awakened. You feel relaxed and receptive to healing. You are at peace.

Other Suggestions for Healing

There are many nurturing activities that can enhance your energy and uplift your mood. I often ask my students to make a list of 20 things they love to do. Some people have a difficult time finding 20 things they enjoy. If that is the case, I ask them to go on a great expedition of discovering what brings joy to their lives. The things on your list can be very simple: walking your dog in the park, working in the garden, listening to uplifting music, or playing a game of golf. I encourage people to do at least one thing they enjoy each day. When you are injured or sick, it is helpful to bring as much enjoyment into your life as possible. Examine the suggestions that follow to see if any speak to you. Make a list for yourself. If there is an activity that your illness or injury prevents you from participating in now, imagine yourself enjoying that activity in your mind.

Above all else, have hope. Hope is one of the strongest healing attributes available to us. Cultivate hope on a daily basis. Give your injured areas love and attention, not criticism or worry. Keep your mind focused on the positive. Have faith.

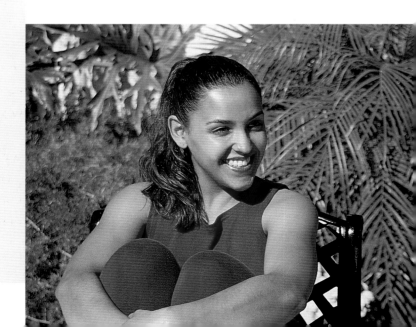

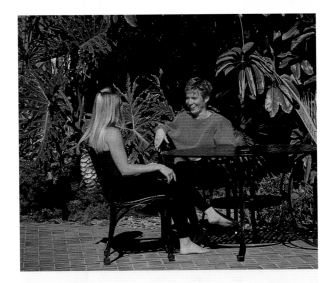

SAMPLE ENJOYMENT LIST

- Listen to uplifting music or chanting.
- Take a warm bath or long hot shower.
- Walk along the ocean, or visualize yourself there.
- Ask a friend to give you a foot massage.
- Listen to interesting books on tape.
- Gaze at a beautiful sunset.
- Surround yourself with art that you love.
- Choose movies and television programs that are inspirational and uplifting, not degrading to the human spirit.
- Get into nature and allow your eyes to absorb the beauty of the environment.
- Spend time with children.
- Have lunch with your best friend.
- Take a watercolor class.
- Join a singing group.
- Spend time in your garden.
- Read an interesting novel.
- Learn a new skill.
- Gently dance to music you love.
- Write down your goals for the future.
- Find things that make you laugh: jokes, stories, movies, memories.
- Feel cozy next to a fire drinking warm herbal tea or soup.

More Stress-Reducing Activities

Sigh: An "ahhh" sound comes out naturally when people sigh. People often sigh when they feel relieved. It is a sign of letting go and a signal to our bodies to do just that. "Ahhh" is also the sound of the heart center. Voicing this sound helps to open the heart center and increase the energy flow through it. When I let out the "ahhh" I like to think of my awe for life. It is a simple practice. When you feel tense, simply give out a sigh. I like to practice it when I am driving. "Ahhh," I am alive. I do not have to hurry. I can enjoy each moment. "Ahhh," the breath and belly release.

Smile: We all know how good it feels when someone smiles at us. A smile is international. It is a warm greeting. Smiles are simple gestures that uplift people and therefore release tension.

Oxygen break: Even five minutes of deep, full breathing or alternate nose breathing is calming, healing, balancing, and relaxing. Oxygen is energy rich, nourishing all the cells in our bodies.

Media vacation: Take a break from watching television and reading the newspaper for a week. We are bombarded with negativity in our media. We hear stories of murders, robberies, violence, and disasters. Television dramas also contain violence and negativity. A week without this negative energy can be healing. Listen to uplifting music instead, or spend more time interacting with loved ones.

Gardening: Spend time gardening, growing plants. Planting seeds and watering and nourishing them is a wonderful metaphor. Plant seeds of healing thoughts as you work in your garden.

We Are All Worthy of Healing

One of the things I discovered when I worked as a substance-abuse counselor at a recovery hospital is that unless alcoholics or addicts felt on a core level that they were worthy of healing, they often sabotaged their recovery. As a counselor I asked myself, "How do you help people to know their worth? How do you teach people to love themselves?" Not easy questions to answer.

What I did find is that when people learn to adapt new lifestyle habits that are self-constructive, rather than self-destructive, they tend to feel better about themselves. Mentally, emotionally, and physiologically we do better when we are nurtured. Sometimes that nurturing has to come from us. And it is important for us to value ourselves enough that we do indeed take the time to enjoy activities that are nurturing for us and that provide self-care.

Our lifestyle choices affect our health. Nutrition; exercise; rest; relationships; finances; work; spiritual practice; play; water consumption; and avoid-ance of alcohol, cigarettes, and drugs—these factors reflect our level of self-care. If we drink 10 cups of coffee a day, we will neutralize our innate ability to heal. Balance and moderation are the keys.

When people feel worthwhile, connected to others, and in harmony with life, they tend to stay well. When emotions are blocked or people feel hopeless or trapped, they often fall ill and may get worse despite the finest treatment. Love and acceptance are essential ingredients for healing. Yet the ability to fully embrace self-love and self-acceptance can be one of life's greatest challenges. We must accept our imperfections and vulnerabilities in order to receive our greatest healing.

Yoga will encourage you to accept where you are and work from there. It is a compassionate, cooperative process rather than a competitive practice. The realization of our own worth becomes evident as we focus our attention on healing.

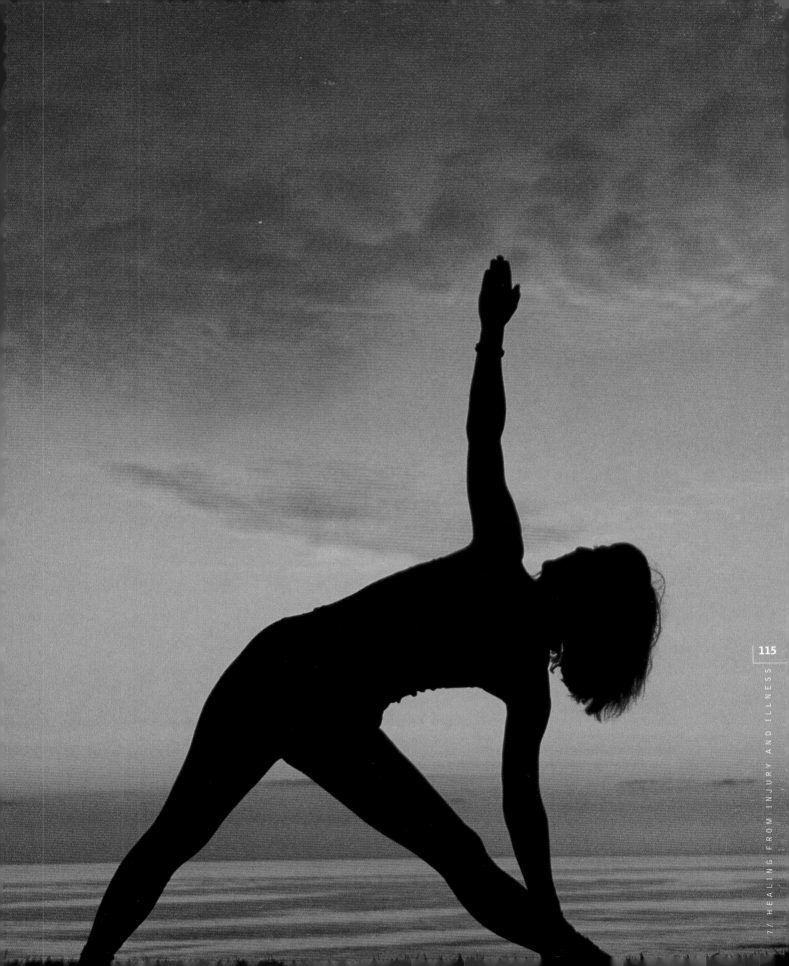

Sample Gentle Yoga Routine for Injury

As you practice the following routine remember to honor your limitations—staying with your inner body wisdom, going to your edge with love and acceptance rather than judgment or discouragement. It is also helpful to allow your healthy twin (the noninjured side of your body) to be the memory friend, showing the way to your potential. Only do what is possible for your particular situation. You can always visualize yourself in the pose if you are unable to move into the position.

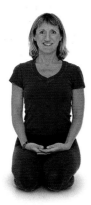

1. The Sitting Mountain (pose 11, page 46). This opens the heart and invites stillness to the body. Use a pillow under your knees or sit on a chair if you need to.

Affirmation:

Serenity comes when I surrender.

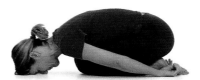

2. Child's Pose (pose 12, page 48). This helps us to feel safe, protected, in a womb of healing energy. Use a pillow or bolster if you have a tight lower back, hips, knees, or ankles.

Affirmation:

I rest in trust and patience.

GENTLE YOGA FOR HEALING

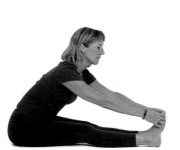

3. Seated Forward Bend (pose 20, page 58). This fosters a sense of calm and letting go, while gently stretching the spine. Place a blanket under your buttocks so you are on your sitting bones.

Affirmation:

I move forward with patience.

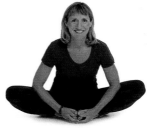

4. The Butterfly (pose 21, page 60). This can be practiced upright or lying down. It opens the knee joints and the hips, so be gentle. You can go into the Inner-Thigh Stretch (pose 22, page 61) for variation. Be careful if you have groin injuries.

Affirmation for The Butterfly:

My spirit is as gentle as a butterfly.

Affirmation for Inner-Thigh Stretch:

Nonresistance gives me peace.

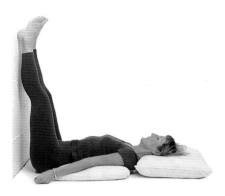

5. Leg Inversion against the Wall (pose 33, page 74). Lace a pillow under your pelvis and lower back for support. This allows you to rest and relax.

Affirmation:

All things are possible.

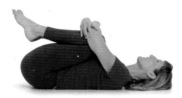

6. Little Boat (pose 26, page 65). After the leg inversion come away from the wall and hug your knees in toward your chest. The Little Boat releases the lower back and lengthens the spine. It is also a form of self-hugging.

Affirmation:

I Trust Myself.

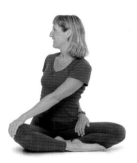

7. Spinal Twist. Do a gentle spinal twist as pictured above, or the knee hug spinal twist on page 69. The spinal twist stretches and relaxes the spine, releasing energy and increasing flexibility.

Affirmation:

I turn in each direction with my heart open.

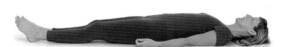

8. Corpse Pose (pose 35, page 78). Final relaxation: Close your eyes, take a deep breath, and let healing energy restore the senses that have been depleted by stress or tension. Visualize healing energy flowing through your entire body. Relax your body, quiet your mind, and soothe your soul.

You may want to use the visualization for pain management with this pose.

9. Meditation practice (page 88–90).

Journal Writing Exercise:

How can you best support your healing process? Are you accepting of your condition or feeling frustrated? What thoughts are the most helpful to focus on? Which friends are the most positive for you to be around? What activities are the most uplifting for your involvement at this time? Write about all the ways you can enhance your healing potential.

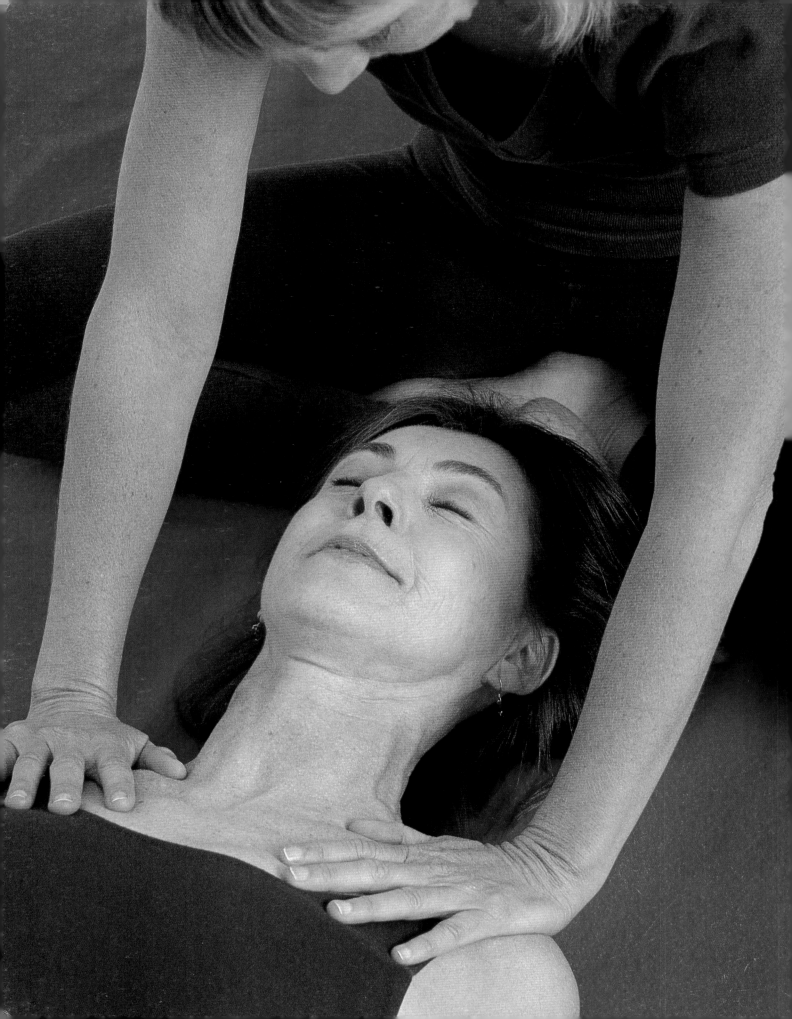

CHAPTER EIGHT

Healing Touch

Therapeutic massage was the first healing modality I studied. I attended massage school when I was 19 years old. Giving massages allowed me to physically feel the difference between tight, contracted, tense muscles in a persons body, and what a muscle feels like when it is relaxed. Chronic tight muscles can actually develop knots of tension that are held in the body. Therapeutic massage helps release the knots of tension, relax the muscles, improve circulation and calm the mind.

Most people do not realize how much tension they are carrying in the neck, shoulders, back, jaw, and other areas throughout their body. Yoga practice teaches people to tune into their body. Massage is another tool for gaining body awareness.

Because I learned massage before I began my study of yoga, I have always incorporated therapeutic massage into my practice. Five-minute shoulder massages are given in partner work just before the period of relaxation. Instructions are given in this chapter. For those who are not comfortable exchanging massage with another person, I recommend self-massage techniques. One of the self-massage practices I suggest using on a daily basis is derived from the Ayurvedic tradition, which is a traditional medical system, developed in India, where yoga also originates. Massage is compatible with yoga as an ancient healing modality that does have roots in India.

Bringing Therapeutic Massage into Your Yoga Practice

As a massage therapist I have witnessed the therapeutic value of touch for many years. Healing touch is another tool for releasing tension in the body. During my yoga classes, I often introduce therapeutic neck and shoulder massage into the practice just before the period of relaxation in the Corpse Pose. I ask people to work in partners, and students learn the value of giving as well as receiving massage. All it takes is a few simple techniques. After just 3–5 minutes of receiving therapeutic massage, the body begins to release tension. The shoulders let go of "the weight of the world" and all those "responsibility knots" begin to dissolve.

Partner Massage

The receiver lies down on his or her back with arms alongside of his or her body. You, the giver, sit above the receiver's head.

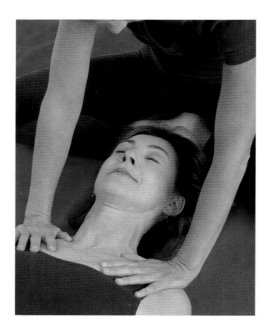

1. Begin by placing your hands on your partner's shoulders and pushing them down toward his or her feet. Place your thumbs under his or her shoulders and press in on the shoulder muscles in circular motions.

2. Now place your hands underneath your partner's neck in a cradle position and gently pull his or her neck to help elongate the spine. You are not pulling up to lift your partner's head; rather you are pulling his or her neck and head away from the body in

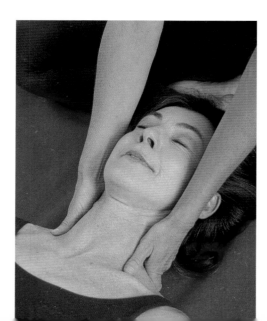

gentle traction. Your hands rest easily along the base of your partner's head. Be sure that you are not resting any fingers on the front of the neck because this will feel uncomfortable for your partner. Never massage the front of the neck. You are working on the back and side neck muscles, which can feel tense.

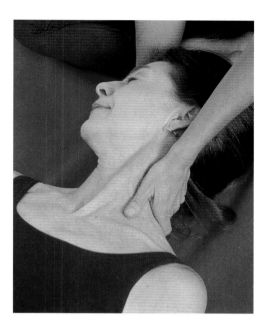

3. Gently turn your partner's head to one side and massage his or her neck muscles, moving your hand along the muscles in circular motions. Always ask for feedback from your partner to make sure the massage feels good. If the pressure is too strong, ease off. It is best to start with light pressure and add more if your partner requests it. Remember that you are massaging the muscles along the spine, not the spine itself.

4. Repeat on the other side.

5. End with your partner's head facing forward and do the gentle neck pull again.

6. Push your partner's shoulders down toward his or her feet.

7. Rub your hands together to generate heat and then place them on your partner's upper chest area to send healing energy into his or her heart center.

Self-Massage Techniques

I pay particular attention to the neck and shoulder area in my yoga classes because the neck and shoulders are often a starting place of back pain and headache. If you learn to keep your shoulders and neck free of tension, you will find it easier to truly let go into relaxation and meditation. Usually when tension begins to appear we ignore it. Rather than ignoring it, learn to self-massage yourself to release tension in your shoulders.

Neck Massage

1. With your fingers together and extended, press in on the sides of your neck next to your spine at the lowest point where the neck and shoulders meet. Press in and rotate your fingers in a circular motion as you continue pressing.

2. Work your way up your neck alongside the spine, pressing and giving a circular massage to the muscles next to the spine.

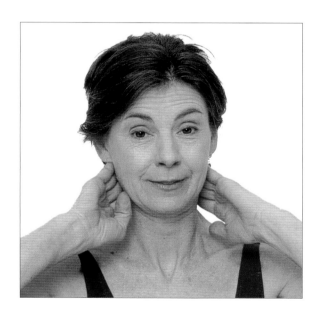

3. At the very base of the spine where your neck meets your head, you will find an indentation, like an opening. Press your fingers into that space and breathe.

4. Then massage your scalp.

Shoulder Massage

1. Place one hand over your opposite shoulder. Push in and then pull your fingers forward over the shoulder. Do this twice.

2. Repeat on the other side.

3. Now take both hands and place them on your shoulders with your fingers on your back, pointing down. Squeeze your shoulders. Release and pull both your hands forward over your shoulders.

4. Release your hands and roll both your shoulders up, down, and around to further release tension.

5. Take a deep breath and let go with a sigh.

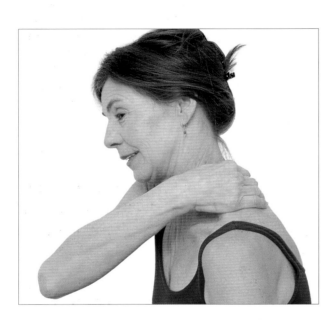

Jaw Massage

Your face can hold a tremendous amount of tension, particularly in the jaw area. I often ask my yoga students how many people grind their teeth; at lease one-third of the class generally raise their hands. Teeth gripping and grinding are signs of tension.

1. Place your fingers at the corners of your jaw, where your mouth opens and shuts, toward your ears. Open and shut your mouth to find the right spot. Press into this point and massage in circular movements.

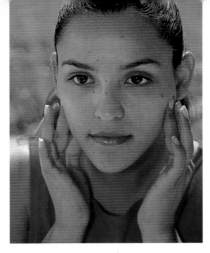

2. Massage all the way down your jaw, pressing your fingers in circular movements.

3. Remind yourself to keep your teeth slightly parted throughout the day so that your jaw learns to stay free rather than clutched.

Forehead Massage and Pull

Whenever I am flooded with thoughts and stuck in my head rather than my heart, I like to do the forehead massage and pull. While using this technique I imagine that I am wiping away all the thoughts.

1. Place your fingers on the center of your forehead and massage it in circular motions all the way across to your temples. Repeat this two or three times.

2. Next, place your thumbs on your temples on the sides of your head and rest your fingertips just above the center of your eyebrows. Slowly pull your hands apart with pressure, so that you are pulling your forehead. Repeat this pull two or three times.

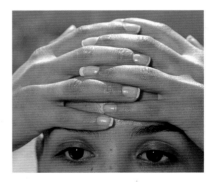

3. Next, place your fingertips along the ridge of your eyebrows and pull your forehead up into your scalp line, running your fingers through your hair.

4. End by bringing your hands down to your heart and taking some deep breaths.

Ayurvedic Self-Massage: to be practiced at home

The self-massage derived from the Ayurvedic tradition is a wonderful way to enhance well being. It can be adapted to your daily schedule taking as long as fifteen minutes or as little as two. It is generally performed before taking a bath or shower in the morning or evening. Oil is used in Ayurvedic massage and considered part of the healing treatment. Different oils are traditionally applied to balance certain conditions. For instance, if you are feeling anxious or have insomnia then a heavier, warmer oil such as sesame or almond is applied with gentle strokes. If you are feeling overheated, irritable, or cranky then you can use an oil with cooling properties such as coconut or olive oil. If you are feeling heavy or sluggish then try a lighter oil such as sunflower or safflower.

Preparing the oil

With Ayurvedic massage the oil is heated. You can slowly heat the oil in a metal pot over the stove, or place it in a plastic container and warm it in a pot of almost boiling water. If you heat it on the stove it must be carefully watched. You can also warm the oil in a plastic container by placing it under hot running tap water for several minutes.

15-minute massage

1. Begin by pouring a tablespoon of warm oil onto the scalp. Cover the entire scalp with small circular strokes, as you would when you shampoo your hair. Give the scalp a vigorous massage. Then move to the face and ears, massaging more gently. Gently massage the temples and backs of the ears.

2. Using both palms of your hands and the fingers, massage a small amount of oil onto the neck, all the way around, and then the shoulders. Massage the arms, using a circular motion at the shoulders and elbows, and long back and forth motions on the upper arms and forearms.

3. Use gentle circular motions as you massage the chest, stomach, and lower abdomen. Ayurveda traditionally advises moving in a clockwise direction. A straight up and down motion can be used over the breastbone. Be sure you have enough oil on your hands to make the massage smooth and soothing.

4. Reach around to massage the back and spine as best you can. Use an up and down motion, spreading the oil. Then massage the legs vigorously up and down to improve circulation, with a circular motion at the ankles and knees. Complete the massage at the feet, covering them with oil, in vigorous movements. Pay extra attention to your toes.

5. Keeping a thin film of oil on the body is considered very beneficial for toning the skin and warming the muscles. Most people like to take a shower or bath after the massage. If you want to enjoy the benefits of leaving the oil on your skin then use a damp, warm washcloth to wash off any excess oil before you get dressed or go to bed. Your skin will have already soaked up much of the oil during the massage.

Two-minute mini-massage

Ayurvedic medicine considers the head and feet to be the most important parts of the body to massage when you are short on time. You will only need two tablespoons of oil.

1. Rub one tablespoon of warm oil into the scalp. Massage the scalp in circular motions. Allow the movement to be vigorous, stimulating the scalp. Then gently massage your forehead from side to side. Gently massage the temples using circular motions, and then gently rub the outsides of the ears. Spend a few seconds massaging the back and front of the neck.

2. With a second tablespoon of oil, massage both feet rubbing them with your palms. Work the oil around the toes with your fingertips. Then vigorously massage the soles of the feet with a back and forth motion using the flat of your palms. Sit quietly for a few seconds to relax and soak in the oil.

Sending Yourself Healing Energy

I have found that simply rubbing my hands together to create heat and energy and then resting them on my tight shoulders or an injured area can be helpful. Take a moment to rub your hands together until you feel them getting warm. Take your hands and place them on any part of your body that needs extra energy. Focus your mind on the energy coming from your hands into your body and take several deep breaths.

Thymus Thump

The thymus thump is helpful in stimulating the thymus gland; the thymus gland helps the immune system to function properly. I suggest that people do the thymus thump everyday and especially on those days when they just do not feel like laughing. We all have days that are unpleasant. On those days we need extra support.

1. Pretend you are Tarzan or Jane and tap your chest in the area around the center of your sternum. You can use your fingers and tap lightly or use your fists like Tarzan did.
2. You can even have fun sounding out an "Ahhhh!" which also releases tension in your throat and jaw.

The Benefits of Giving and Receiving Hugs

Most people know how wonderful it is to be greeted by a warm hug from someone you care about. Hugs communicate affection and compassion and help people to be less guarded and more open in their hearts. This brief exchange of energy between two people is another form of healing touch. If a person is feeling down a hug can sometimes be the best remedy. Hugs are also given in times of celebration. If there are people in your life that you feel comfortable hugging then let that be one of your practices on a daily basis. It especially feels good to give hugs to children that we love.

Hugging Yourself

If you are not involved with people that you feel comfortable hugging, then give yourself a hug. Fold your arms around yourself and squeeze. Breathe deeply and know that you are loved. It's that simple.

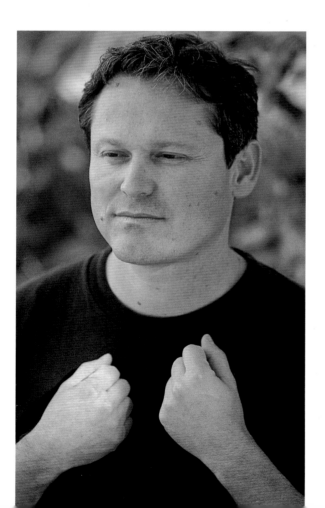

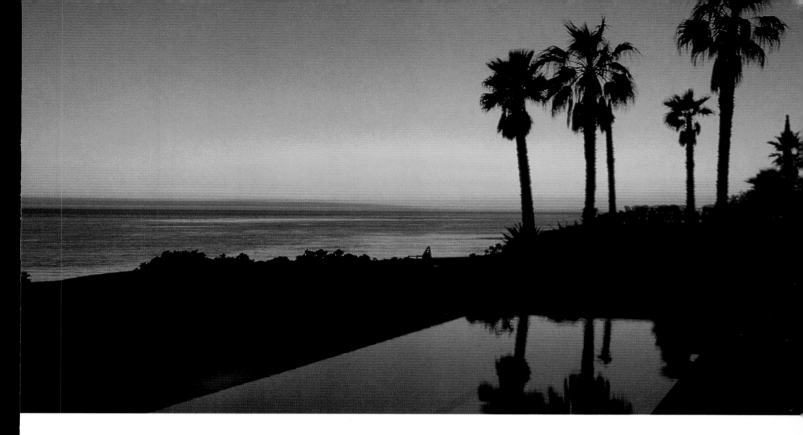

Healing Touch Visualization

1. Lie down on your back in a comfortable position on the floor. Make sure you are resting on a blanket or mat so that your body is comfortable. Place your arms along the sides of your body with palms faced up. Close your eyes. Breathe deeply and slowly, allowing your body to sink into the floor.

2. Push your shoulders down toward your feet. Make sure your teeth are slightly parted so that your jaw is relaxed. Roll your head gently from side to side, and then relax your neck and head. Take another deep breath. Feel the energy with your body as you are resting in this position. Notice if there is any tightness or tension in your body at this time. Is there any pain in your body? If you find any area that feels uncomfortable don't judge it, just notice it. Continue to breathe deeply.

3. Now imagine that a healing angel is placing her hands on the area of your body that is feeling tight, uncomfortable, or painful. If you did not find any area that was uncomfortable then imagine that the angel is placing her hands on your chest, which is the location of the heart center. You can feel the hands of the angel gently touching your body, sending you healing energy. Feel the warmth of energy going into your body, helping it to relax and melt away all tightness and pain. The angel is sending

you love and light through her hands to the area of your body that needs healing. Breathe in and receive the light and healing energy that this angel sends you through her hands.

4. Continue to rest as long as it feels comfortable.

Journal exercise

Notice if there is any area in your body that needs healing attention and write about the sensations you feel in that area. Is there tightness? Do you feel any contraction, soreness or pain? Describe how your energy feels in that area of your body, and what thoughts you have regarding the situation. Then take a few moments to send yourself healing energy (as described in this chapter), or use one of the self-massage techniques. If you can't reach the area with your hands then place them nearby. Use your intention to send yourself healing, calming energy with your hands. Write about what happens when you do this. Describe how it feels to send yourself healing energy or self massage. What changes occur, if any?

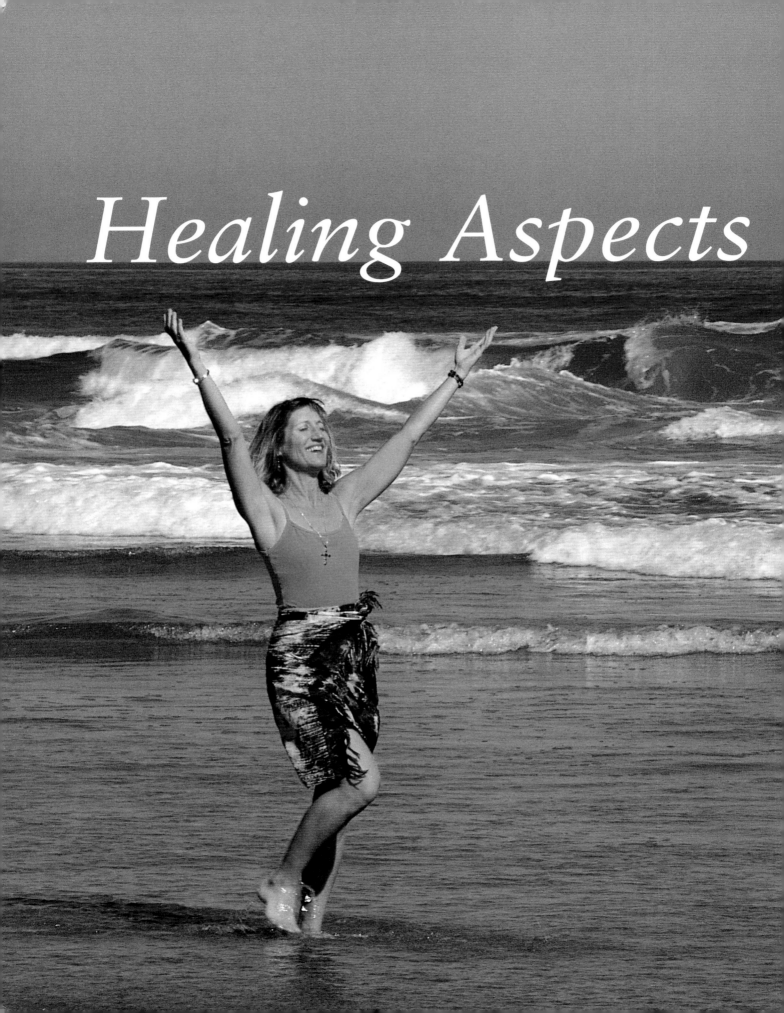

Healing Aspects

# of Nature

Yoga can be practiced indoors or out. I have always done both. Although spending time in nature is not a requirement for yoga practice, it is extremely healing and beneficial. I often combine yoga practice with hiking in the mountains, swimming in warm oceans, meditation by a stream, or traveling to sacred power spots where the Earth's magnetic healing energy is more evident.

In this chapter, I will mention a few places that I have found to be quite powerful. But the more important message is that you can enhance your energy by spending time in nature wherever you live. Even if you live in a city, you can bring aspects of nature into your life by creating simple gardens or having plants in your home and by going to nearby city parks where you have access to lawns and walking trails.

Nature is filled with energy. The air we breathe, the earth beneath us, the trees, the plants, the rivers, the oceans, the mountains—all contain positive life energy. Spending time in nature enhances our own energy, particularly if we bring our

awareness to the energy that surrounds us and is available to us.

Spending time in nature is especially important in people's lives when they are dominated by technology. Computers, televisions, microwaves, cell phones, beepers, and driving in traffic are examples of our modern lifestyle choices that can be taxing to our physical energy over time. Our bodies are not built to sit all day staring at a computer screen or television, or to drive in traffic. Although technology gives us many advantages, it does take its toll on our energy and well-being. I am amazed at how disconnected some people are from the Earth's energy. Walking on pavement, driving in cars, living in high rises, sitting at computers, and eating processed food are all activities that keep us disconnected from the natural rhythm of the Earth. Ultimately we get our food and nourishment from the Earth. Nature sustains us.

To counter the effects of our high-tech fast-paced lifestyle, I recommend spending time in nature often. It is a simple practice, yet very effective. The

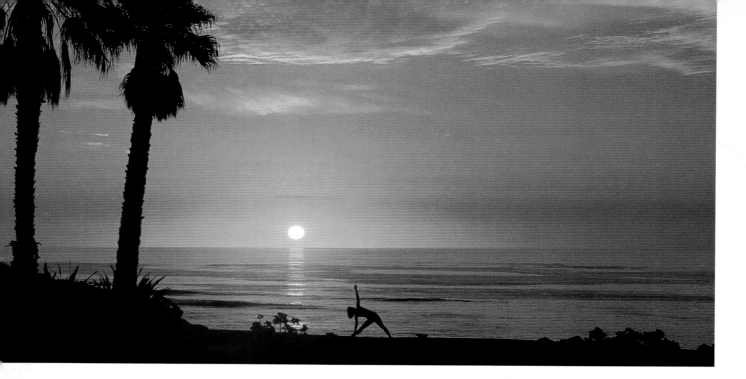

frequency of the Earth's energy is calming and balancing to human beings.

There are several ways to enhance your connection with nature. The first is to consciously bring your body in touch with the Earth. Take time to go barefoot on the Earth. Take your shoes off when you are on a grassy area, dirt, or sand at the beach. If you can, lie down on the Earth and practice breathing with her. The Earth is a live being that nourishes us. Feel the Earth beneath you, supporting you completely. Notice if your life has you constantly walking on pavement or cement. Find a place where you can walk on the Earth.

Another way to bring nature into your life is through plants and gardens. If you live where you cannot have a garden, then buy some indoor plants. Plants give off positive oxygen. They offer a vitality for our living environments. If you do have room to create a garden, then the tasks of planting seeds, tending your garden, watering, and

nurturing growth can become a metaphor for your own growth in life. Planting a garden is a healing activity.

Water is a third element of nature that can be brought into your life. If you are lucky enough to live near warm oceans, rivers, lakes, or creeks, then take the time to swim or at least walk through knee-high water as often as possible. Swimming pools and hot tubs with chlorine are not as ideal, but do still offer the feeling of washing away static energy and tension. Swimming is wonderful exercise and soaking in a hot tub can be quite soothing to muscle tension. Simple fountains in your home or ponds and birdbaths in your yard can also have a calming effect. The element of water is soothing to the soul.

Finally, getting outdoors in fresh air is invigorating. It is not healthy to be indoors all day long. This is especially true for those people who work in offices without windows, where there is florescent lighting and a lack of ventilation, which can be draining to our energy. Take time each day to be outdoors. If you live in an area with poor air quality, attempt to get away to the mountains or ocean as often as possible. Practice yoga breathing exercises daily to enhance your energy.

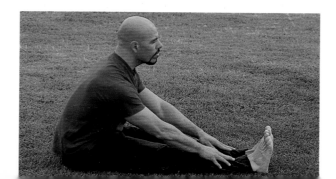

Powerful Places on Earth to Practice Yoga

There are many wonderful places on Earth that are ideal for yoga practice. In my book *Yoga Vacations: A Guide to International Yoga Retreats* (Avalon Travel Publishing), I list over 100 yoga vacation opportunities. Yoga vacations are often held in natural settings. I have been fortunate to travel to many of the places in my book, so I know how wonderful it can be to practice yoga next to the ocean, in the mountains, by a river, near a hot springs, or in the desert. What is ideal about yoga is that it can be practiced anywhere. After reading my book, people often ask me, "Which is your favorite yoga vacation?" Answering that question is like comparing oranges to apples. I do not have a favorite. Each one has its own unique flavor. I love practicing yoga in the mountains, and I love being by the ocean. The desert has a beauty of its own. Here are just a few suggestions of the many opportunities available on Earth for being close to nature and practicing yoga.

Yoga by the ocean: The Yucatan next to the Caribbean Sea is a wonderful place to go to do yoga. The color of the aqua-blue ocean next to the white sandy beaches will make you feel like you are in a postcard. The sand is warm and inviting for yoga practice, followed by a swim. Being able to visit the ancient Mayan ruins is an added benefit; some people claim that the ruins are power spots for healing and growth.

Yoga in the mountains: Mt. Shasta in northern California is another great place for yoga practitioners. Shasta has been referred to as the Healing Mountain for years by spiritual seekers. I recommend camping there in the summer, hiking the mountain, and enjoying yoga practice.

Yoga in the desert: Sedona, Arizona, is also a great choice. As you drive through the Arizona desert toward Sedona, your eyes will be awed by the striking appearance of Sedona's red rocks. The vortex energy of the red rocks is said to be quite powerful and attracts tourists from all over the world. When I was there, I hiked to all the vortex energy spots and practiced yoga right on the side of the red-rock mountains.

Yoga on an island: Hawaii is a magical place. Any of the islands are ideal for yoga practice. The fresh fruit, fragrant flowers, warm ocean, and gor-

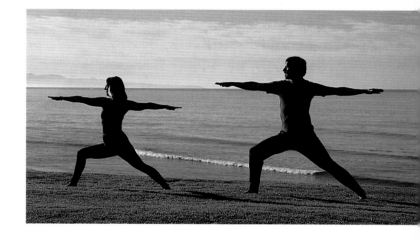

geous sunsets make the islands a paradise for experiencing nature. Each island is said to have its own special energy. The one I am most familiar with is the Big Island, which has the volcanic energy of eruption and creation of new earth. The power of death (letting go) and rebirth can be felt on this island.

These are just a few suggestions. Of course there are several more oceans, mountains, deserts, and islands to choose from. You can also practice yoga next to the snow in a warm cozy cabin, next to a river or lake, by a natural hot springs, or in a meadow of wild flowers—the possibilities are endless. Any place that is surrounded by nature will enhance your experience.

Journal Writing Exercise: How often do you spend time worrying and fretting? Where do you feel the safest in your life? Who do you feel the safest with? How can you remind yourself to have trust and faith when the storms of stress hit your life?

Sacred Mountain

Imagine that you are sitting on top of a high sacred mountain. It has been a long, slow climb and now that you have finally reached your destination you feel exhilarated with a sense of accomplishment. You sit down on the top of the mountain and relax. You feel the mountain beneath you, supporting you completely as you breathe in the fresh invigorating mountain air. There is nowhere you have to go right now. There is nothing you have to do but simply breathe and be. Breathe and be.

From the mountain you see clear views all around you. And this reminds you to view your

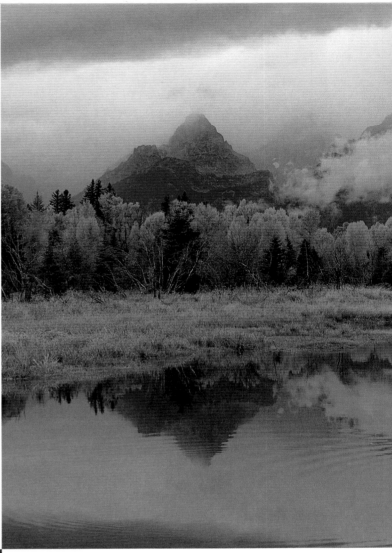

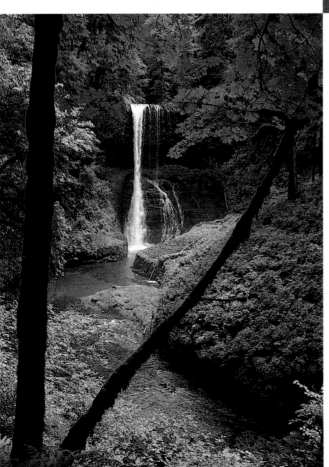

own life from a distance, as well, rather than being caught up in the day-to-day circumstances of your life. You see that your life has been a series of experiences that have provided opportunities for growth and sharing love. There have been various relationships, roles that you have performed, lessons that you have learned, and themes for growth that weave together to create the tapestry of your life. Now, as you view your life from a distance, look at your present circumstances.

Journal Writing Exercise: What is the theme of your life at this time? How do you most need to grow?

Yoga and Swimming with Dolphins

Spending time in nature is healing and uplifting. Interacting with natural creatures can *also* be healing. One of the blessings I have had is the experience of combining my yoga practice with swimming with dolphins.

One of the annual yoga retreats I offer is held on the Big Island of Hawaii near Kealakekua Bay where Hawaiian Spinner dolphins can be seen swimming in the bay. I have had the opportunity to swim with these dolphins and so have my retreat participants. Because they are wild, we never touch the dolphins, feed them, or chase after them. We always take great care to respect the dolphins, allowing them to approach us if they choose to. Amazingly, the dolphins in this bay are highly interactive and like to swim near humans.

As a student of yoga, I have found the dolphins to be wonderful examples of living in a loving community. Ananda, the first place I ever studied yoga, is a community named after the Sanskrit word for joy. Truly, the feeling of joy is one of the great gifts these dolphins offer. Swimming in ocean water next to a pod of wild dolphins (I call them wild because they are not contained, but a better word may be free), you can observe how playful and caring they are with one another. I think the dolphins have much to teach us humans.

Dolphins swim together in pods. Sometimes an entire pod of dolphins swims in a spread formation in a quiet and methodical way. They breathe together and dive together in groups of eight or twelve. It is as if an energy surrounds them as they swim together in unison—and this is what the word "yoga" means: yoke, union, unity, community. As they swim in continuous communication with one another, it is as if they share the mindset: "we are one." Remembering that we are all connected, "we are one" is a very good yoga practice. Dolphin energy demonstrates how to live in harmony with one another, how to cooperate with one another, and how to form loving communities.

During my yoga retreats, the participants come together too as a community of yoga practitioners. What is wonderful about these planned vacations is that we have quality time with one another. Each person is a gift to the group. We practice breathing exercises together, stretching, visualization, massage, and meditation. We eat our meals together and share our personal stories. As we relax our bodies, relax our minds, and open our hearts, we find more patience, acceptance, and tolerance for our differences, as well as more peace and joy in sharing this time.

One of the things I noticed when several dolphins were swimming quite close to me was that many of the dolphins have wounds and scars from life in the ocean. Some have round indentation marks from sharks, and many have scar lines that look like scrapes. It reminded me that all creatures have their scars to bear. And that many of our scars, lines, wrinkles, and what we call flaws are really our affirmations of survival, strength, and vulnerability in being alive.

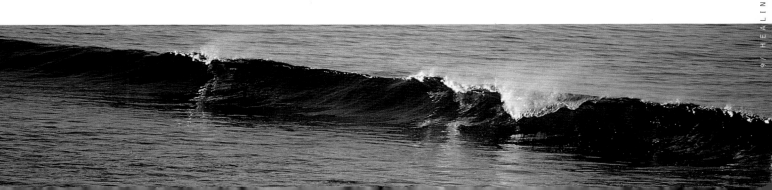

Another interesting trait of the dolphins is that they are conscious breathers. Unlike humans, dolphins must remember to breathe. Although they live in the water, they breathe air. Several dolphins will swim up to the surface of the water together, breathe in unison, and then swim back down. I cannot help but think that their breaths are fully accessed, unlike humans, who often breathe quickly and shallowly. Conscious, complete breathing is another yoga practice. Try taking a deep full breath in unison with another person. Breathing together is another example of the dolphins' unity with one another.

After the experience of swimming with dolphins, people often report a feeling of positive well-being.

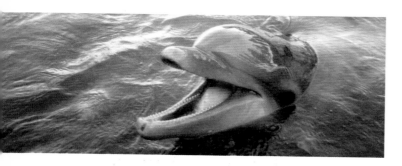

A shift occurs from lower consciousness (marked by fear and separateness and by the tension that accompanies these states) to a higher consciousness (marked by clarity and joy).

I believe that part of the reason we humans feel so good around dolphins is because of the sound frequencies that dolphins send out, the dolphins' sonar. In the water, you can hear their sounds long before you see the dolphins. They sound like clicks and whistles. Dolphins use sonar echolocation, seeing the world with ultrasound. This is, in essence, vibrational medicine. Medical science is discovering that ultrasound frequencies, although inaudible to humans, nevertheless have a calming and pleasurable effect on us, possibly triggering the release of endorphins.

After swimming with these glorious creatures I did some research to discover more about how

their sounds may affect humans. Captive-dolphin studies in Florida, in which the brain waves of participants were measured by electroencephalograph (EEG), show that more than 80% of the participants who had a dolphin encounter experienced a shift from beta brain waves (indicative of high activity) prior to the encounter to alpha and theta brain waves (indicative of a deeply peaceful state similar to meditation).

I am not in favor of keeping dolphins captive or of supporting their captivity by swimming with them. You do not even need to swim with wild dolphins to receive the benefits I am describing. You can also reach this peaceful alpha-theta brain wave state through yoga practice and meditation. It is possible that listening to recorded sounds of dolphins also may be helpful. At the end of this section is a dolphin visualization that I have written and some sources for dolphin recordings.

During my retreats in Hawaii, yoga practice helps us prepare for the dolphin encounter by moving our spines in fluid positions that are not part of our usual earthbound stance. Our breathing exercises help clear stagnant energy held within our bodies. Yoga also helps us to be in and stay in the moment. Trying too hard and wanting the dolphin encounter too desperately may actually hinder a person's chances of having a dolphin swim near him or her. Giving up the struggle and allowing things to unfold has profound implications for our health and life direction. As creatures of the Earth, moving into the element of water invites openness to the immediacy of intuition, feeling, sound, movement, and vibration. We bring this experience back to our earth life and create our own pod, living within community and unconditional love.

At the time of this writing, there is some controversy about the impact that swimming with dolphins in their natural environment has on them. One of the problems is that people want to swim with the dolphins in areas where the animals come to rest, mate, and give birth. The truth is that we do not know whether or not we are disturbing their behavior patterns. It is obvious to me that the dolphins do enjoy interacting with humans. But I also feel that it is important to regard these creatures with great respect.

If you have the opportunity to swim with wild dolphins, know that you are in their territory, not yours. Do not overstay your welcome. Educate yourself about the dolphins' habits and their habitats. In writing this section, it is not my intention to encourage more people to swim with dolphins but rather to awaken the yoga unity consciousness that often emerges when people swim with dolphins. I encourage you to create your own pod of humans with whom you can live, play, and work in harmony. Practice conscious breathing, yoga movement, meditating, listening to healing sounds, spending time in water, accepting your wounds and scars, regarding others with love, and embracing the mindset that we are not separate—we are one.

Dolphin Visualization

Imagine that you are swimming in the warm blue waters of an ocean bay. You are swimming in a bay that is calm and easy to glide through. You are breathing through a snorkel fin in a slow, easy manner as you enjoy all the sights you see through your mask. The water is clear and everything is visible.

As you continue swimming further out toward the ocean, you begin to hear the faint sounds of dolphins, which are even further out in the sea. You can hear their clicks and whistles, which resonate through the water to your ears. You follow their sounds, swimming easily, until you are guided to the place in the bay where the dolphins are swimming together in pods.

Imagine yourself surrounded by dolphins. Pods of eight and twelve dolphins circle around you, swim next to you, and some of them even look you in the eye. You are not afraid because there is an under-

SOURCES FOR DOLPHIN RECORDINGS

Celebration of the Hawaiian Spinner Dolphin
Magical Island Sounds
74-5602 Alapa Street, Suite 340
Kailua-Kona, HI 96740
1-800-341-3680; 808-328-9530
www.magicisle.com

Guardians of Atlantis
Solitudes Ltd.
1131A Leslie Street, Suite 500
Toronto, ON M3C 3L8
Canada
www.solitudes.com

Eye Within Studios
P.O. Box 192, captain cook, HI 9670 USA
email: contact@eyewithin.com
www.eyewithin.com

standing between you. You are here to exchange friendship. You do not touch or chase the dolphins, but simply follow their lead as they swim with you and offer their heartfelt communication. These silvery angels are gentle, loving creatures. And they somehow manage to transfer that love to you.

What joy you feel to be among these glorious creatures who allow you to swim with them! You observe how playful they are with one another. You watch the dolphins swim together and then leap into the air as if to demonstrate their joy and enthusiasm.

Imagine yourself joining the dolphins as they slip back beneath the surface of the ocean, where suddenly, all is calm. You breathe easily as you glide through the water in the serene embrace of a gentle current, surrounded by an azure glow, and a ceiling of sunlight glistening down through the water. Earthly thoughts disappear in this ethereal realm that is both infinity and a peaceful womb. You are safe. You are loved.

Journal Exercise: Write down experiences in your life that have given you joy. Note how many of these experiences are related to being part of nature or being with ones you love. How do you express your joy and enthusiasm? How often do you feel joy in your life?

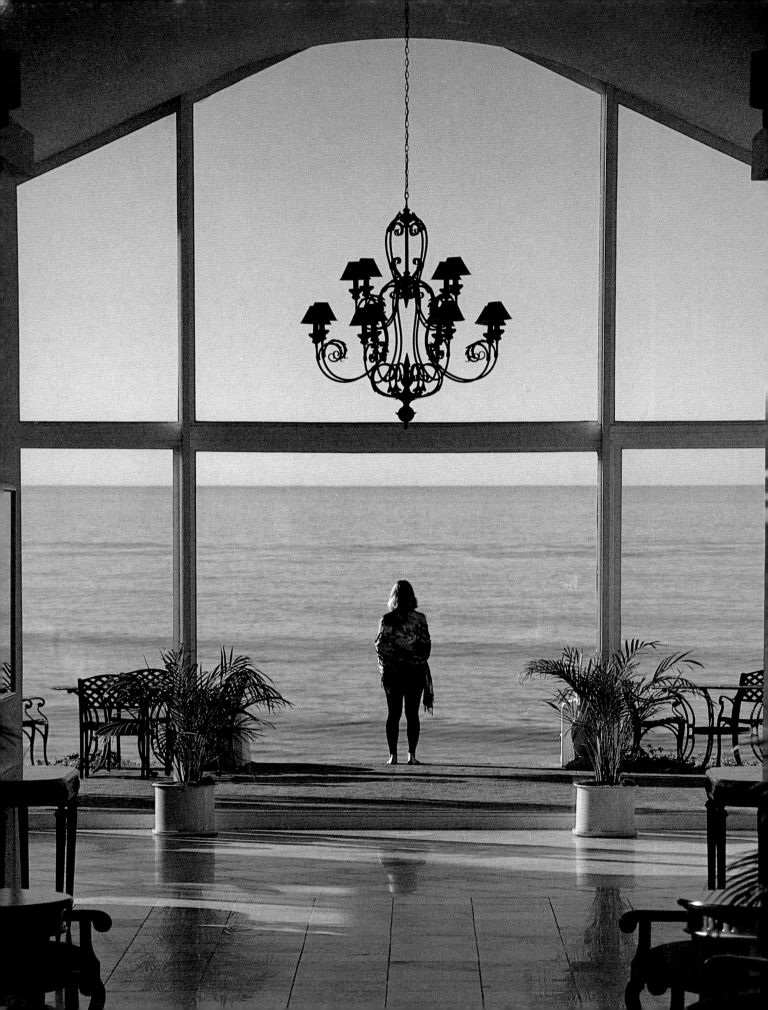

CHAPTER TEN

Yoga Is a Lifetime Journey

Gentle yoga can be your lifetime friend. You can practice it at any age.

Start where you are with your body and take it slowly one day at a time. The idea is not to become perfect or to compete with others but rather to develop a routine that works positively for you.

As you become familiar with the yoga practices and incorporate them into your life, the benefits you receive will help you to understand that yoga is a lifetime practice. When you practice hatha yoga, your body is strong and flexible and you have more energy and less stress. If you stop the routine for a while you will notice the difference: more stiffness, less energy, less flexibility, and more stress.

Developing new habits is not always easy. It takes conscious effort. It takes willingness and patience. Often I approach my yoga practice "just for today." Just for today, I will remember to breathe deeply. Just for today, I will think positively about myself and others. Just for today,

I will spend time stretching my body. Just for today, I will eat nutritious food. Just for today, I will allow myself to relax. Just for today, I will meditate.

And, of course, the "just for todays" add up to create a healthy lifestyle in which I am taking care of myself. One of the most important benefits of yoga practice is that it helps me achieve a stillness of mind. When my mind is still, I can focus on the present moment rather than worrying about the future or thinking about the past. This is especially valuable to me when I am stressed.

Finding peace is a great reward. One of my favorite quotations is from the great yogi Paramahansa Yogananda: "Peace emanates from the soul and is the sacred inner environment in which true happiness unfolds."

Practicing *gentle yoga for healing mind, body, spirit* has helped to bring more peace and happiness into my life. May you, too, find peace on this planet, in this lifetime, in this moment. Blessings on your journey.

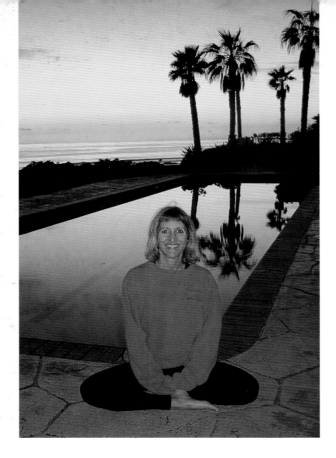

About the Author

Annalisa Cunningham has a Master of Arts degree in counseling. She has been a certified hatha yoga instructor, massage therapist, a Reike practitioner, and counselor for more than 25 years.

She specializes in gentle hatha yoga for healing and stress-reduction lifestyle training. Combining her love of yoga, health, and travel, Annalisa offers annual yoga vacations in Mexico, Hawaii, Costa Rica, and Northern California. She is the author of several books, and writes articles for numerous popular magazines.

Annalisa enjoys connecting with people and welcomes contact from her readers. To find out more about her vacations, order her books and CDs, or to contact Annalisa please go to her website: www.openingheartjourneys.com

Supplemental Books and CDs by Annalisa Cunningham

If you would like to order any of the following products please go to website: www.openingheartjourneys.com or send an email to *annalisa@openingheartjourneys.com*

Books:

Stretch and Surrender: A Guide to Yoga for People in Recovery
$16.95 (plus tax & shipping.)

Yoga Vacations: A Guide to International Yoga Retreats
$16.95 (plus tax & shipping.)

Spa Vacations: Your Guide to Healing Centers and Retreats
$16.95 (plus tax & shipping.)

Healing Addiction with Yoga - A Yoga Program for People in 12 Step Recovery Findhorn Press, England September 2004

CDs:

Stretch and Surrender
40 minute yoga class with affirmations and relaxation/visualization

Chakra Meditation
30 minute healing meditation on the chakras using visualization with color and affirmations

Nature Visualizations
4 relaxation/visualization scripts set in nature, 10 minutes each, designed for a stress-release break during your day

Each CD is $15.00 (plus tax & shipping)

Video:

Yoga Vacations and Getaways
Hour-long video features 8 vacations
$29.00 (plus tax & shipping.)

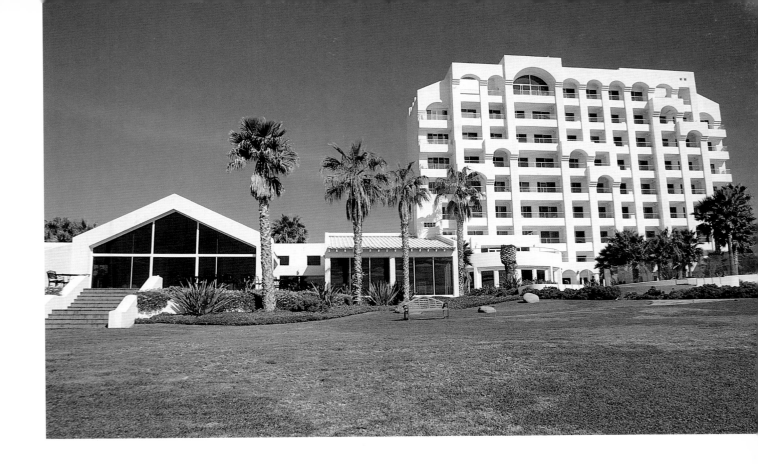

On Sanoviv

Many of the photos in this book were taken at Sanoviv Medical Institute in Baja California, Mexico. I learned about Sanoviv while researching another book I wrote, *Spa Vacations: Your Guide To Healing Centers & Retreats*. After spending a week at Sanoviv I was so impressed with the beauty of the place that I decided it would be an ideal environment for the photos in *Gentle Yoga For Healing*. I'd like to thank Dr. Myron Wentz for his kind permission to take these photos at Sanoviv and for his warm hospitality.

Sanoviv Medical Institute offers personalized healing programs, which combine conventional and alternative healthcare therapies for people suffering from cancer, degenerative diseases, depression, and for those who simply want to improve their overall health. Programs include nutrition and detoxification, extensive diagnostic testing and assessment, spa and fitness therapies, psycho/spiritual counseling, daily meditation, and biological dentistry.

For information:
1-800-SANOVIV or *www.sanoviv.com*

Suggested Reading

Diet and Health

Ornish, Dean. *Dr. Dean Ornish's Program for Reversing Heart Disease.* New York: Random House, 1990.

Ornish, Dean. *Everyday Cooking with Dr. Dean Ornish: 150 Easy, Low Fat, High Flavor Recipes.* New York: Harper Collins, 1997.

Weil, Andrew. *Natural Health, Natural Medicine.* Boston: Houghton Mifflin Co. 1995.

Weil, Andrew. *Spontaneous Healing.* New York: Knopf, 1995.

Mair, Nancy. *The Intimate Vegetarian* (a cookbook). Nevada City CA: Crystal Clarity Publishers, 2000.

McCord, Blanch Agassy. *The Expanding Light Cookbook.* Nevada City, CA: Crystal Clarity Publishers, 2000.

Mind/Body Medicine

Benson, Herbert. *The Relaxation Response.* New York: Avon, 1994.

Borysenko, Joan Ph.D. and Miroslav Borysenko, Ph.D. *The Power of the Mind to Heal.* Carson, Ca: Hay House, 1994.

Borysenko, Joan. *Fire in the Soul: A New Psychology of Spiritual Optimism.* New York: Warner Books, 1994

Chopra, Deepak, M.S. *Quantum Healing: Exploring the Frontiers of Mind-Body Medicine.* New York: Bantam Doubleday Dell, 1990.

Cousins, Norman. *Head First: The Biology of Hope and the Healing Power of the Human Spirit.* New York: Penguin, 1990.

Dossey, Larry, MD. *Prayer is Good Medicine: How to Reap the Healing Benefits of Prayer.* San Francisco: Harper San Francisco, 1996.

Benson, Herbert, MD. *Timeless Healing: the Power and Biology of Belief.* New York: Simon & Schuster, 1996.

Hay, Louise. *You Can Heal Your Life.* Carlsbad, CA: Hay House, 1999.

McGarey, Gladys. *The Physician Within.* Deerfield Beech FL: Health Communications, 1997.

Pert, Candace. *Molecules of Emotion.* New York: Scribners, 1997.

Shealy, Norman. *Miracles Do Happen: A Physician's Experience with Alternative Medicine.* Rockport, MA: Element books, 1996.

Siegel, Bernie, M.D. *Love, Medicine and Miracles: Lessons Learned about Self-Healing from a Surgeon's Experience with Exceptional Patients.* New York: HarperCollins, 1990.

Simon, David, M.D. *Return to Wholeness: Embracing Body, Mind, and Spirit in the Face of Cancer.* New York: John Wiley & Sons, 1999.

Kabat-Zinn, Jon. *Full Catastrophe Living: Using the Wisdom of Your Body and Mind to Face Stress, Pain and Illness.* New York: Delta Books (Dell Publishing), 1990.

Women's Health

Northrup, Christine. *Women's Bodies, Woman's Wisdom: Creating Physical and Emotional Health and Healing.* New York: Bantam Doubleday Dell, 1994.

Weed, Susan S. *Menopausal Years The Wise Woman Way: Alternative Approaches for Women 30–90.* New York: Ash Tree Publishing, 1992.

Yoga

Devi, Nischala Joy. *The Healing Path of Yoga.* New York: Three Rivers Press, 2000.

Suggested Listening:
CDs and Autocassettes

Feuerstein, Georg, Ph.D and Larry Payne, Ph.D. *Yoga for Dummies.* New York: Hungry Minds, Inc., 1999.

Francina, Suza. *The New Yoga for People over 50.* Deerfield Beech FL: Health Communications, 1997.

Kraftsow, Gary. *Yoga For Wellness.* New York: Penguin, 1999.

Miller, Richard. *The Therapeutic Application of Yoga on Sciatica - Article and Workbook.* Anahata Publications, P.O. Box 1673, Sebastopol, CA 95473

Scaravelli, Vanda. *Awakening the Spine.* San Francisco: HarperCollinsPublishers, San Francisco, 1991

Lasater, Judith. *Relax and Renew: Restful Yoga for Stressful Times.* Berkeley, CA: Rodmell Press, 1995.

Schiffman, Erich. *Yoga: The Spirit and Practice of Moving into Stillness.* New York: Pocket Books, 1996

Shivapremananda, Swami. *Yoga for Stress Relief.* New York: Random House, 1997.

Meditation

Bodian, Stephan. *Meditation For Dummies.* Foster City, CA: IDG Books Worldwide Inc. 1998.

Fontana, David, Ph.D. *Learn to Meditate: A Practical Guide to Self-Discovery and Fulfillment.* San Francisco: Chronicle Books, 1999.

Healthy Travel

Cunningham, Annalisa. *Yoga Vacations: A Guide to International Yoga Retreats.* New Mexico: John Muir Publications, 1999.

Cunningham, Annalisa. *Spa Vacations: Your Guide to Healing Centers and Retreats.* CA: Avalon Travel Publishers, 2001.

Infinite Awakening Yoga Nidra with Richard Miller
A complete program of deep relaxation, intensive self-inquiry and profound meditation that reveals our true nature as radiant presence.
Anahata Publications, P.O. Box 1673, Sebastopol, CA 95473, www.nondual.com

Non-Dual Meditation with Richard Miller
Guided meditation recorded during a live workshop using body sensing and breath awareness to reveal our true nature as radiant presence.
Anahata Publications, P.O. Box 1673, Sebastopol, CA 95473, www.nondual.com

Breathing for Life with Richard Miller
A five-part series that teaches how to use the breath for deep relaxation and meditative self-inquiry in order to reveal true nature as unqualified presence. Anahata Publications, P.O. Box 1673, Sebastopol, CA 95473, www.nondual.com

Deep Relaxation with Nishala Joy Devi
Provides a complete 30-minute guided relaxation with gentle flute accompaniment. Abundant Well-Being P.O. Box 346 Fairfax, CA 94978-0346 www.abundantwellbeing.com

Sojourn to Healing: Creative Imagery and Visualization with Nischala Joy Devi
Explains the theory of imagery and visualization. Provides two complete 15-minute guided imagery sessions with relaxing flute music. Abundant Well-Being P.O. Box 346 Fairfax, CA 94978-0346 www.abundantwellbeing.com www.abundantwell-being.com

Dynamic Stillness Meditation Guidance with Nishala Joy Devi
Explains the theory of meditation with basic, simple and varied meditation techniques. Instruction for beginners as well as those wanting to deepen their inner stillness. Abundant Well-Being P.O. Box 346 Fairfax, CA 94978-0346 www.abundantwell-being.com

Relax, Move & Heal with Nischala Joy Devi
Gentle guidance through movement, relaxation, breathing, imagery and meditation. Abundant Well-Being P.O. Box 346 Fairfax, CA 94978-0346 www.abundantwellbeing.com

Index

GENTLE YOGA FOR HEALING